Growing Pains

THE DEVELOPMENT OF CHILDREN'S MENTAL HEALTH SERVICES IN SASKATCHEWAN

BY TERRY RUSSELL

ISBN 978-0-9919109-0-8

The cover drawing is by Terry's granddaughter,
Hayley Thomson

Typeset at SpicaBookDesign in Book Antiqua

Printed and bound with www.createspace.com

Foreword

Terry Russell died in the winter of 2007. At the time this manuscript was with a publisher who eventually declined to publish the book because the potential market was small. I have now attempted to update parts of it to reflect recent changes and have added a final chapter on Regina Child and Youth Services today. The clinic, begun with a staff of four in the basement of the Regina General Hospital, is now in a purpose-built facility with a staff of seventy-five. Terry would have been so pleased!

Terry was a man with strongly-held views, dogged determination and a life-long commitment to children. His work was always principle-based. He was very active locally, provincially and nationally in the world of services to children. One of my enduring memories of him was of the many nights he sat at the dining room table surrounded by papers, an ashtray, often a beer in hand, writing funding proposals, strategizing how to get additional positions, drafting begging memos to central office asking for more staff, for policies and for them to pay attention to children or working on one of the many national initiatives he was so often involved in. He was in great demand as a public speaker and the children and I were well used to meeting new people who, when they realized our relationship to Terry would tell us of hearing him speak and about some family incident that he had used to illustrate a point. The stories were always kind and often funny so we didn't mind.

In 1968 Terry established the first specialized mental health program for children, youth and families in southern Saskatchewan. During the Saskatchewan years he was an Adjunct Professor of Psychology at the University of Regina and was the first civilian instructor in the Royal Canadian Mounted Police training academy. He sat on the board of the Canadian Council on Children and Youth and chaired a national task force which published *Admittance Restricted: The child as citizen in Canada*. He was founding co-chairperson of the Board of Management of the Canadian Youth Foundation and was recognized nationally as an expert on child and youth mental health policy and was frequently called upon to speak at national forums and events.

In 1986 he became Director of Child and Youth Mental Health Services for the British Columbia Ministry of Health with responsibility to develop and implement a province-wide network of specialized mental health services based in an interdisciplinary system of care model.

The book tells the story of how children's services developed – building upon the systems, structures and expertise established over the decades of Canadian and Saskatchewan history. Surveying the history of the province from the 1880s onward, he describes a population first of all concerned primarily with survival but quickly beginning to create the support services communities need – schools, hospitals and other social services. There was cooperative action and an early recognition of the need to prioritize development. Children were rarely a priority in the early days. Terry identifies what was required to change that. Throughout the development of health services there were common forces – public servants with a vision and the operational abilities to bring their vision to reality, politicians with the will to work with and support this and pressure from the community. When all three of these are in play, much can and does happen.

Terry also lays out a set of principles that should underlie service provision – and that do form the foundation of the children's programs that now operate in Saskatchewan.

Laura Carment, a long-time colleague of Terry and also a former director of Regina Child and Youth Services has continued to be an invaluable ally, writer and editor as this document has been updated. The errors, however, are mine alone.

Sharon Russell
May 2013

Preface

Much has been written about the history of mental health services for adults in Saskatchewan. Most of it focuses on the closure of mental hospitals and the development of community psychiatry in regional centres throughout the province. However, the parallel story about the development of mental health services for children and youth has not, until now, been written. In fact, I am not aware of a written history of the development of mental health services for youngsters in any province. This book describes the development of mental health services for children and youth in Saskatchewan in the context of the Canadian experience.

A significant aspect of a modern mental health service for children is that it is an interdisciplinary system involving psychology, psychiatry, psychiatric nursing, nursing, speech therapy, occupational therapy and social work. The other child-serving systems tend to be dominated by a single profession – for example, teachers in schools and social workers in child welfare and youth justice. However, the main lesson of the last fifty years for all who work with children is the need for the systems to understand each other and find ways to work together on behalf of youngsters and their families. It is hoped that this work will assist in this process of collaboration by helping all to understand better the mental health approach – an approach that is always multi-disciplinary and at best interdisciplinary.

It is only in the last fifty years that there has been a concerted focus on the development of mental health services for youngsters in Canada. It is timely to record how these services were developed in one jurisdiction and how they have changed over time. The methodology used to produce this book involved research in the Saskatchewan Archives and Legislative Library. The cooperation of my colleagues who were involved through the years has been freely given and I thank them for their assistance. Of necessity the end product will be a personal account as there are all too few primary documents in these collections. Much of the information that forms the basis of the story is from my personal files. I intend to lodge these with the Saskatchewan Archives at the end of this project. I accept responsibility for any errors or misrepresentations that readers may find in the text.

In telling the story of the development of mental health services for children and youth in Saskatchewan a number of analytic frameworks are used to illustrate the complexities. The first part addresses the questions: What is mental health and what do we mean by mental health services in Canada? A discussion of the two predominant and often competing models for the provision of mental health services for children and youth – the child guidance model and the child psychiatry model – will be illustrated by comparing the services provided in the province with a focus on service organization and management. The child's place in Canadian society and law – how children are viewed by society – and the consequences for service development and delivery provide the broad context for understanding.

This is followed by a description of the overall service delivery system – health, education, social and justice services – for youngsters and the interrelationships among the systems. Then the document describes the early history of health services in Saskatchewan with special attention paid to two streams, child health services and psychiatric services. The uneven growth of services through to the end of the 1960s sets the stage for the changes to come.

Next there is a case history of the development of Regina

Child and Youth Services. In each of the Health Regions in Saskatchewan the development of mental health services for children was shaped by the needs and characteristics of the area but all were based upon the same principles as described herein.

This is followed by the recommendations of the Review of Child and Youth Health that was completed in celebration of the International Year of the Child. The final section discusses the factors that have influenced the changes that have been made in services to children in the last fifty years.

Lastly, a comment on the title that I chose – Growing Pains. Children often experience growing pains. As you will find out by reading this book, mental health services for children and youth in Saskatchewan experienced growing pains too. Indeed, growing pains are a natural part of achieving maturity – not always fun but a necessary part of life.

Acknowledgments

This project began as an account of the development of the first free standing mental health program for children and youth in the city, Regina Child and Youth Services. Plans were made to celebrate the 37th anniversary of the program in 2005 which was also Saskatchewan's Centennial year. Two of my friends and former colleagues, Laura Carment and Mary Jean Martin, both of whom were also former directors of the program offered lots of support, old files to dig through and their eagle eyes on early drafts. My thanks to them both for I never would have completed the project without their help. Like Topsy, the book just grew – first to describe the early history of mental health services in Saskatchewan and later to provide a national context to aid the reader to better understand mental health services for children and youth.

My greatest help in completing the project was provided by my wife, Sharon Russell. Her constant encouragement pushed me to complete the book when it seemed I never would. More importantly, her skills as an editor made sense out of my often uneven prose. Without her help the book would not have been finished.

Lastly, I'd like to acknowledge my children – Paul, Sarah and Kate. Over the years, they have taught me a lot. In the early days of Regina Child and Youth Services, before they started school they were most intrigued by the question: Why I was the boss at my work? Before I could answer their question they answered it themselves. "I guess you got there first" was the first response. The answer given by my second child was "I guess you're the boss because you are not too bossy and not too nice; just a little bit bossy and a little bit nice". My third child was not old enough to talk. I am sure she would have been equally supportive. This book is about children, their mental health and wellbeing. In the years to come I hope that everyone will listen to children and learn from them as I have been fortunate to be able to do.

Table of Contents

1

Understanding Mental Health and Mental Health Services

Children are society's most valuable asset and society's primary goal must be to ensure that they thrive. The health, physical and mental, of children and youth is of critical importance as it represents an investment in the future health of Canada. Families and communities share the responsibility for children – to ensure that they have the resources to promote health, well-being and optimal development.

It is increasingly clear that attention to child development is one of the most serious challenges facing society in the twenty-first century and that this includes the need to promote optimal mental health for children and youth and to ensure that specialized services are available to resolve the problems of those who have mental disorders.

It is often too late when children and youth with mental problems and mental disorders are identified and referred into the system. Early interventions can help these children and youth lead normal productive healthy lives and save the costs that would otherwise be incurred if it becomes necessary to provide them with social services throughout their adult lives.

Senator Allen Kirby's Standing Senate Committee on Social Affairs, Science and Technology Out of the Shadows at Last says:

> "The Committee is deeply concerned about the capability of the mental health system to respond to the needs of children and youth. Fragmentation coupled with under-funding, a shortage of mental health professionals, and a failure to involve younger people and their families in long-term treatment solutions, has resulted in the delayed application of inadequate treatment interventions. . . . a much greater investment in children's mental health is required if it is to shed its label as the 'orphan's orphan' within the health care system"[1]

All jurisdictions in Canada are faced with the problems of providing adequate services to meet the mental health needs of youngsters.

Historically, mental health policies and programs have largely focused on the treatment of the adult population; consequently, services for the young have developed slowly and as an adjunct to programs for adults.

WHAT IS MENTAL HEALTH

To understand the issues involved in developing services for young people it is helpful to have definitions and a framework to think about the concepts and some knowledge of the historical models that have been used in Canada to develop specialized services. It is also useful to consider the principles that form the basis for program policy and that would be useful in the future to inform the development of mental health legislation for children and youth. And finally the social and legal context and history that govern the provision of services in Canada is a critical piece of the picture.

The definition of health in this document is from the Constitution of the World Health Organization, "Health is a state of complete physical, mental and social well-being and not merely the absence of disease . . . Healthy development of the child is of basic importance; the ability to live harmoniously in a changing total environment is essential." Health is a dynamic relationship between the person and his/her environment. Narrowing the focus to mental health, it ". . . is the capacity of the individual, the group and the environment to interact with one another in ways that promote subjective well-being, the optimal development and use of mental abilities (cognitive, affective and relational), the achievement of individual and collective goals consistent with justice and the attainment and preservation of conditions of fundamental equality."

Furthermore, "No longer is mental health conceived of as an individual trait, such as physical fitness; rather, it is regarded as a resource consisting of the energy, strengths and abilities of the individual interacting effectively with those of the group and with opportunities and influences in the environment."[2]

Narrowing the focus even further, two terms are frequently used – mental disorder and a mental health problem. A mental disorder is defined as ". . . a recognized, medically diagnosable illness that results in the significant impairment of an individual's cognitive, affective or relational abilities." On the other hand, a mental health problem is defined as "a disruption in the interactions between the individual, the group and the environment."[3] Mental health problems may result from factors within the individual (physical or mental illness, inadequate coping skills) or unfavourable environmental conditions. The important point is that mental disorder is not the only factor determining mental health. It is a single element within a much larger set of interconnected factors. In planning for the development of services both factors need to be taken into account.

The critical point to be made is that neither mental disorder factors nor negative environmental factors alone account for the mental health status of children and youth. Rather the mental health status of children and youth is the dynamic interaction between vulnerability (mental disorder) and risk (environmental factors).

Mental disorders constitute the most important group of health problems that children suffer in terms of the number of children affected and the degree of impairment involved.[4] International research shows that the overall community prevalence for mental disorders in children and youth is about 14%.[5] This means that more than one million children in Canada suffer from mental health conditions that affect their daily lives.

The most common mental health problem among children and youth is anxiety. It is followed by conduct, attention and depressive disorders. Eighty percent of all psychiatric disorders emerge in adolescence and are the single most common illness that onset in the adolescent age group.[6] Research indicates that at any given time approximately one in seven Canadian children and youth under the age of 19 are likely to have a serious mental disorder that impacts their development and ability to participate in common adolescent activities.[7] Sadly, only one in five Canadian children who need mental health services currently receive them[8].

RISK FACTORS INFLUENCE MENTAL HEALTH

Negative internal factors such as illness or coping ability and negative external factors like family dysfunction or community tensions influence the mental health of youngsters. The primary risk factors that affect children's mental health follow:

- **Relationship bonds** – Their formation and maturation are critical to child and adolescent development. A failure to develop close attachments or a disruption of relationships through separation, death, divorce or any other factor may result in mental health problems.

- **Emotional attachment** - Mental health problems arise when youngsters experience emotions that overwhelm them and manifest in excessive or prolonged fears, sadness, irrationality, anger or unacceptable behavior.

- **Cultural attitudes, beliefs and values** determine how youngsters think and act. When there is a discrepancy between the culture of the family and the broader community, problems of an anti-social nature often arise.

- **Intellectual aptitude, styles of thinking and educational achievement** are strong influences on how children think of themselves and as a consequence on their behaviour. Early school failure often results in problems of self- image that last throughout life.

- **Physical and sensory development or abnormalities and medical problems** influence mental health. Children with developmental delays, brain damage, chronic disease and sensory disorders are at increased risk of maladjustment to society's expectations.

- **Socio-economic factors** such as poverty, poor housing, excessive mobility and high unemployment often result in youngsters being deprived of love, intellectual and emotional experience and meaningful human relationships that contribute to the development of poor mental health.[9]

Additionally, developmental factors play a significant role in the mental health of children and youth. Many children do not 'grow out of a problem' as is often believed. Rather, they grow out of the childhood symptoms while the underlying problems remain into adulthood.

SERVICE DELIVERY MODELS

There are two predominant models described in the literature which provide mental health services to children and youth – the child guidance clinic model and the child psychiatry model. Both are valuable but neither is sufficient alone to meet the mental health needs of young people. Often some characteristics of both models exist in a service.

The child guidance clinic model is based in the community and the staffing is multi-disciplinary. The clinics provide assessment and treatment and focus predominantly on consulting to other community agencies such as schools, family services and child welfare agencies. In this way, the specialized services of mental health professionals can be multiplied throughout the community. Child guidance clinics tend to see a larger number of children for shorter periods of time. The focus of the child guidance model is to improve the mental health of all children and youth. Jones[10] in *Taming the Troublesome Child* describes the beginnings of the child guidance movement in rescuing wayward youth from the effects of poverty and mental retardation. Lourie[11] shows how the modern community mental health approach in the United States grew out of the tradition of child guidance. The most comprehensive description of the American community mental health approach is found in *The Handbook of Child and Adolescent Systems of Care,* edited by Pumariega and Winters[12].

The child psychiatry model is based in the hospital and provides both inpatient and outpatient services but with the major expenditure of effort and resources focused on inpatient care. In its simplest form, this model removes the child from family and community to cure the problem in the child. When the youngster leaves the inpatient care unit there may be insufficient services available to maintain the gains that have been made. This model tends to see fewer children for longer or more intense periods of time. The focus of the child psychiatry model is to provide services to a child or youth with a mental disorder.

Programs that are built with the goal of improving the mental health of children and youth are not developed in the same manner as programs focused on meeting the needs of youngsters with mental or emotional disturbances. Neither model is sufficient to meet the needs of all children, both models need to work together with the service providers in the community if the mental health needs of children and youth are to be met. Practitioners trained and experienced in one model do not necessarily understand or appreciate the other. Rather than work together there is often competition for scarce resources as child guidance clinics and child psychiatry units are frequently administered and funded by separate organizations.

GUIDING PRINCIPLES FOR POLICY AND LEGISLATION

A discussion of the principles upon which services are built will result in a better understanding of mental health services. In Canada there has been no singular overall approach to the development of mental health legislation or policy or the evaluation of services for children and youth.

In all provinces, child and youth mental health needs fall under the jurisdiction of general mental health legislation that has been developed based only on the needs of adults with mental disorders. Alberta and Ontario have additional pieces of legislation that were introduced to deal with specific problems related to children and youth. Since 1976 Ontario has had legislation that allows funding for certain types of services to be provided[13] and in 1985 Alberta passed legislation governing the provision of secure treatment for youth as part of its child protection legislation.[14] Neither of these acts provides a comprehensive approach to legislation for children's mental health.

During the 1980s there were two national processes that had an impact on services for young people. First was a federal-provincial review of mental health legislation the *Uniform Mental Health Act*[15] and, secondly under the Criminal Code a national review of the legislative status of mentally disordered offenders. Neither of these reviews recognized the special problems of children and youth even though they are affected by the legislation. Other federal legislation, specifically *The Young Offenders Act 1984*[16] and provincial legislation governing schools in all provinces recognizes the need to address the special need of youngsters with emotional and behavioural problems.

Admittance Restricted: The Child as Citizen in Canada[17]

proposed four principles as the basis for the relationship between children, their families and society. These principles form the basis on which to develop mental health legislation and policy:

- Human rights are indivisible and are not to be parceled out to different segments of society at different times and under different circumstances.

- Support for the family is the single most important manner by which society can see to the rights of children.

- Equality of opportunity can best be achieved through social policy legislation that addresses equity for children and youth and supports parental responsibility.

- Individuality of interest means that society must take care to ensure that the interests of the child remain uppermost when the matter of rights is the focus.

Within this broad conceptual framework of rights for children and youth Russell[18] developed a set of principles to be used in developing social policy and legislation to meet the mental health needs of children and youth.

- Federal-Provincial consultation is needed to ensure common expectations across provinces, legislative standardization, research and technology transfer and adequate professional training standards.

- Interdepartmental/ministry planning is essential given the division of governments into separate administrative units. Duplications are wasteful and discontinuities are troublesome to consumers.

- Cooperative area structures are needed to account for the differences in boundaries among departments/ministries responsible for services. Cooperation needs to be dependent upon authorized mechanisms and agreements not individual good will.

- Regulations and policy consistent with legislation are required to ensure appropriateness and effectiveness of the services that are based in the legislation.

- Program standards and evaluation based on predetermined expectations for outcomes that ensure equity, accessibility, training and qualifications of staff are necessary for all funded programs.

- Additional costs of special services including factors such as community size, population density and relative wealth must be taken into account by funding authorities.

- A comprehensive continuum of services including prevention, rehabilitation and treatment should be available and coordinated both horizontally and vertically.

- Early intervention and developmentally appropriate services require special policy and designated funding to ensure their availability.

- A priority for youngsters with severe and chronic problems to have access to early, specialized and intensive services and easy access across service delivery systems is required.

- The family as the basic social unit when serving youngsters needs to be recognized in policy and practice.

- Recognition of the transitional status of youth gradually becoming more responsible for their own care and needs should be legislated and followed in practice.

- Normal social integration with peers, family and community opportunities including respect for cultural and linguistic needs is important to the mental health of children and youth and needs to be recognized in policy and practice.

- A least restrictive intervention priority must be the basis of clinical and program decisions.

- Informed consent policy must be clearly stated so that the young person and the family are knowledgeable about the diagnosis and treatment options. A youngster who is not deemed old enough to consent to treatment should receive the same rights to review as an involuntary patient.

- Involuntary care and treatment should be provided in consultation with the child welfare service. There should be no overriding authority to coerce treatment beyond that available through the Mental Health Act. Age appropriate criteria for involuntary care should be established and monitored.

- Due process safeguards and advocacy opportunities should be a part of the mandate of the mental health service and necessary supports built into the system of care.

This presentation of guiding principles that should inform a mental health service for children and youth provides a starting point for legislative and policy development. They are included in this first chapter because they provide the broader social context in which mental health services have developed in Canada. These principles help to understand the potential breadth of impact that mental health services for children and youth have in the community.

THE SOCIAL AND LEGAL CONTEXT
GOVERNING SERVICES

To understand what mental health means and to describe mental health services for children and youth it is important to understand the place of young people in Canadian society. That is, what is the social and legal context that governs how children are viewed in law in Canada? This view of children informs the basis of the development of the services that have an impact on them. For the most part, the law defines children as all those below the age of consent which is 18 or 19 years depending upon the jurisdiction. So, children in this context includes children and youth.

The governance and organization of services to children and youth in Canada has evolved in an historical socio-legal context. Canada was created in 1867 by the passage in the British Parliament of the *British North America Act*.[19] This remained Canada's main constitutional document until 1982 when the Canadian Constitution[20] was proclaimed, incorporating the Charter of Rights and Freedoms and retaining, for the most part, the allocation of powers between the federal and provincial levels of government.

The *BNA Act* had not a single reference to children. In the allocation of powers between the federal government and the provinces, areas of concern for children were primarily allocated to the provinces. The federal government maintained authority to make laws about marriage and divorce, citizenship and the criminal law. As well, laws pertaining to First Nations children are in the federal domain. Provincial legislatures have jurisdiction over education, health care and child welfare and are predominant as measured by the constitutional allocation of powers, the quantity of legislation, the administration of courts and services and financial responsibility. Mental Health Services are in the provincial sphere of responsibility.[21]

The allocation of powers between federal and provincial governments had implications for children. The result has been that the provinces are predominant in governing matters related to youngsters by most significant measures: constitutional allocation of powers, quantity of legislation, administration of services and courts and financial responsibility.

The provincial predominance in laws concerning children is somewhat different in Quebec because it is governed by the *Civil Code*. Elsewhere in Canada the legal system is derived from British common law and is based on custom and usage, confirmed by the decisions of judges and distinct from statute law. Judicial decisions often known as case law are used as precedents for arguments in subsequent litigation. Civil law, on the other hand, rests on a theoretical discussion of legal principles, leading to their application in each like case. Decisions in Quebec civil courts often consist of a general discussion of a rule of law, of its scope and limitations, followed by a judgment of the case in point that is settled either by a principle or an exception to a principle. In considering strategies for changes to the laws affecting children it is necessary to consider the application of both civil law and common law.

The relationship between the federal and provincial governments while dynamic is often uneasy. The federal influence in child and family policy is mainly through the transfer of payments to provinces of federally collected taxes and through legislation in areas of federal domain. Regional or provincial economic and social disparity is a constant issue in Canada. With the predominant responsibility in the provincial sphere and a tradition that respects provincial autonomy, disparities frequently exist. A large variety of methods have been used over the years to discourage provincial economic and social disparities and to encourage comparability of services across the provinces. The tradition is to maintain provincial autonomy and over the years the federal role has lessened.[22]

Canada has developed various methods of dealing with the development, disparity and inconsistency of law and social policy. The Council of First Ministers brings together the governing political leaders on a regular basis for discussion leading to policy agreement. The model is repeated, for example, with Councils of Ministers of Health, Social Services, and

Justice. As well, there are corresponding networks of public servants who meet as Federal/Provincial/Territorial committees and advisory structures concerned with addressing social, economic and legal policy issues.

Another successful model is used by the Council of Attorneys General which has established a mechanism called the Uniformity Commissioners, experts in the law, who meet on a regular basis to debate, draft and adopt by resolution uniform measures which provincial legislatures are then able to enact as they choose.

Because education is totally a provincial responsibility the provincial ministers of education meet on a regular basis without federal representation as the Council of Ministers of Education. There is a corresponding network of public servant committees and working groups. The tradition in Canada is for public education to be managed locally by elected school board officials, similar to a municipal form of government.

As provincial authority is paramount in social programs a common approach is for one province to develop a new model or program which is observed by other provinces and, if successful, adopted by other provinces and often by the Government of Canada. In this way, Saskatchewan successfully pioneered universal hospital insurance in 1946 and medical care in 1964. Within a few years, the federal government developed a national medicare scheme. This is yet another manner in which the provinces deal with the development and disparity in social programs.

The Canada Health Act[23] governs the provision of insured hospital and physician payments in all provinces. In the past hospitals were frequently run as nonprofit or charitable societies with boards of governors elected from the community at large. In recent years, many of the provinces have developed a system of regional health services wherein all health services in an area are administered by a single regional health board. In all provinces the provincial government through Departments of Health is responsible for overseeing the provision and payment of health care. Governments fund medical care, develop standards and guidelines for care and are increasingly involved in ensuring that effective utilization management is in place to control costs and that there is an effective and efficient delivery of health care.

In the 1960s the provinces and the federal government jointly signed the Canada Assistance Act[24] which legislated a framework for the delivery of a wide range of social programs, including income assistance, child welfare and services for people with mental handicaps on a cost-shared basis. Throughout the decade of the sixties common approaches to the provision of laws and services were enacted by the provinces.

This had a major impact in shaping new program development as provinces used creative approaches to ensuring that new programs were eligible for cost sharing.

By the 1990s the federal government had become concerned about the large fiscal deficit and began making major budget cuts. One result of this was that federal participation in legislating social programs and providing cost-sharing for health care, social programs including post secondary education decreased significantly. For the provinces this meant much less federal money. However provinces have traditionally expressed the desire for greater independence and flexibility in managing resources and subsequent programs. Social programs are now funded based in an agreement, The Canada Health and Social Transfer Program[25] rather than the more prescriptive approach taken in the past.

Through these mechanisms, questions of social policy and equity are debated and consensus achieved. The confederation remains one of mutual influence rather than one of central power. The Canadian tradition is participatory and oriented to consensus rather than top-down. The major responsibility for law and social policy for children and youth and the delivery of services remains in the hands of the provinces, closer to home, where the effect can be most direct.

MENTAL HEALTH LEGISLATION FOR
CHILDREN AND YOUTH

The *Mental Health Act* in each province or territory governs mental health services for children and youth. In the main, mental health legislation governs the manner in which people with mental disorders receive voluntary or involuntary services with the majority of emphasis in legislation placed on inpatient care. However, in two provinces, Ontario and Alberta, there is legislation specific to young people. It is generally true that where services are mandated by legislation, the services are viewed by the government and the general public as more legitimate than services with no such mandate. Consequently, the lack of a legislative mandate is often seen as a deficit.

The Ontario legislation dates from 1970 and has been updated several times over the years. The pattern of services developed in Ontario prior to this time had resulted in a wide range of facilities of uneven quality, supervision, funding and distribution throughout the province. The legislation ensures that all special treatment programs for children and youth that are funded by government shall be designated, licensed and appropriately funded. All designated centres are also designated psychiatric facilities under the *Mental Health Act* and are eligible to receive operating grants and capital assistance. A significant feature of the Ontario program is that no child admitted to a licensed centre shall be denied treatment because of inability to pay. Licensing of centres implies that they will be inspected on a regular basis and will be expected to maintain provincial standards.

The *Ontario Mental Health Centres*[26] *Act* is just that, an Act regarding mental health centres. It is not a broadly based act regarding mental health nor does it speak to the mental health needs of children and youth except through making operational grants, licensing and inspecting facilities. Nevertheless, it is a step in legitimizing services that has not been replicated by other provinces.

The Alberta legislation is the responsibility of the child protection service and provides for a youth who is deemed by a psychiatrist or psychologist to have a mental disorder to be held in custody for a time-limited assessment. The legislative mechanism for this custodial assessment is the *Child and Family Services Act*[27] rather than their mental health legislation. British Columbia has passed similar legislation but to date it has not been proclaimed and has not been used.

2

The Context – the National
Scene to 1985

SOCIAL POLICY ADVOCACY FOR CHILDREN AND
YOUTH IN CANADA

Canada has a long tradition of local community action on behalf of the young. Saskatchewan was typical. In the early part of the twentieth century as the province was settled, local groups built schools and hired teachers, recruited doctors and built hospitals. Pioneers understood and practiced the adage: "It takes a village to raise a child." While in the 1990s we reinvented the concepts of mutual aid and community development in the name of health promotion, we are only beginning a new cycle that was at the centre of the community for our pioneering forefathers and foremothers.

As will be seen throughout this document, three factors are key to the social change that has resulted in improving mental health services – government commitment, visionary professionals and community advocates.

Prior to the second world war the service delivery system

was a mixture of local community agencies, often organized and run by charitable and church groups, and government operated, specialized institutional services. For example, specialized facilities for blind children were developed as national residential schools and many provinces including Saskatchewan ran provincial schools for the deaf. Children with physical and mental disabilities including mental illness were sent to provincial hospitals and institutions. It was common for youngsters with physical and mental disabilities and disorders to grow to maturity, live and die in a care facility.

In the years following the war the federal government and the provinces gradually increased their emphasis on child-centred and family social policy. However it is important to note that there has never been a committed politician providing concerted leadership on behalf of children's mental health. There is no national or provincial organization in Canada standing up for, speaking out about and advocating for the mental health needs of the young. Groups of parents of children with specific mental health problems, for example, autism spectrum disorders and learning disabilities have been successful on behalf of their children locally, provincially and nationally. The parent movement has been concerned with specific disorders rather than the broader field of mental health.

Through the 1970s, the British Columbia Law Reform Commission on Children's and Family Law[28] and the Saskatchewan Law Reform Commission report on Children's Maintenance[29] were among the provincial actions that highlighted a new appreciation of the needs and rights of children. The federal government also played an active role through house and senate standing committees, law reform and special commissions such as the Committee on Sexual Offences Against Children[30] which debated the problems of abused and neglected children. The result was a revolution in care provisions.

Parallel to government action, national advocacy bodies were growing in importance. The Canadian Association for the Mentally Retarded, the Canadian Association for

Children with Learning Disabilities, the Canadian Council on Children and Youth, the Canadian Child Health Institute, and the Canadian Youth Policy Institute were among those that provided information and advocated on behalf of the young. These organizations were important partners in Canada's contribution to the International Year of the Child in 1979 and the International Year of Youth in 1984. It was during this time that a balance began to be achieved between the social policy needs of the child with special needs and social policy based on the personal, social and economic inequities and opportunities of the children and their parents.

This focus on social policy advocacy on behalf of children, youth and their families continued through the 1990s with Canada and Pakistan taking the lead role at the United Nations in the adoption of the United Nations Declaration of the Rights of the Child.[31] Another theme that has focused the attention of social policy makers in Canada is the population health movement's attention on the determinants of health rather than merely trying to come to terms with the sequelae of disease and disorder.

It is key to remember that children and youth have no direct voice in social policy debates. The needs of the young are expressed by others in the debate on social policy. No matter how benevolent the authority that speaks on behalf of children and youth the interpretations and decisions usually reflect the reality and represent the interests of adults rather than children.

This traditional position is summed up by the Law Reform Commission of Saskatchewan in their 1976 background paper, Children's Maintenance:

> "Many of our laws pertaining to children, although perhaps well-intentioned, have been excessively protective. This has led to a reconsideration of the traditional legal emphasis on sheltering the child. The detrimental effect that paternalism has had on the status of women may provide striking support for this emerging view." [32]

There is no doubt that we need to shift our perspective regarding children. Children have been viewed as the property of their parents to be treated by them as they saw fit. Historically, the state has only intervened in special or extreme circumstances to protect children. It is only recently that children are beginning to be viewed as persons in society with individual interests that need to be protected in the same manner as the interests of adults. The child person – the child as citizen – are emerging concepts that have not been fully articulated. Human rights are indivisible. They are not to be parceled out to various segments of society at different times and under different circumstances. What is different about children is not the rights to which they should be entitled but the mechanisms through which those rights should be exercised. Those who join the public debate on social policy on behalf of children and those who make decisions on behalf of an individual child must do so with care so that the interests of children are foremost.

ACTIVITIES THAT SHAPED THE CHANGING VIEW OF CHILDREN IN CANADA

The sections that follow summarize many of the major activities of the last fifty years in Canada that when viewed together portray the changing views of children in Canadian society and the approaches that have been taken to address the mental health needs of young people in Canada.

CANADIAN CONFERENCES ON CHILDREN

A powerful force for change during the 1950s and 1960s was a series of major child-focused forums called The Canadian Conferences on Children. These conferences provided an opportunity for concerned citizens, mainly professionals, to meet and debate the needs of youngsters.

In 1964 at the last conference those in attendance agreed to the formation of the Commission on Emotional and Learning Disorders in Children (CELDIC) and established the Canadian

Council on Children and Youth to act as a national organization concerned with social policy and advocacy.

THE CANADIAN COUNCIL ON CHILDREN AND YOUTH

Through the 1960s the Council acted as the host of the CELDIC research and public participation activity. The Council was active during the next twenty years and was involved in a host of social planning activities on behalf of children and youth. The work of the Council included the creation of the National Task Force on the Child as Citizen in Canada[33] as a lead up to the International Year of the Child. It was also responsible for a report *Children and Culture in Canada*[34] submitted to the Federal Cultural Policy Review Committee, a preliminary analysis of the report of the Committee on Sexual Offenses to Children[35] including a media kit that sparked local action and ensured media attention, and the development of the Canadian Youth Foundation as Canada's legacy to the International Year of Youth.

Each of these activities involved advocacy on behalf of young people and the involvement of youth in planning and working towards solution was always an important consideration.

In 1975 the Council established the Task Force on the Child as Citizen in Canada. It was composed of professionals in child and youth services primarily those involved in researching or interpreting the law in practice. The Task Force report *Admittance Restricted: The Child as Citizen in Canada*[36] provided a baseline from which to understand the place of children in Canadian law recognizing that they have a gradually developing capacity to understand and express their citizenship and participate in society.

In the law, "nonadults" – children – are those citizens between the ages of birth and eighteen or nineteen depending upon the jurisdiction and the individual laws. In this section the term children is used to mean citizens below the age of majority.

The most powerful description of the place of children in Canadian society is provided in the report *Admittance Restricted: The Child as Citizen in Canada.* [37]

The report states that children "make up about a third of our population. Yet, they remain largely invisible in social policy and planning. They do not have the right to vote and they cannot influence policy". From the point of view of the law, children are primarily a provincial responsibility. The Task Force outlined a reasoned approach to the rights of children under the law recognizing their diminished but gradually increasing responsibilities. Three key elements were identified for society to consider when considering the rights of children: supports for the family; equality of opportunity; and individuality of interest.

A quote from Mr. Justice Edson Haines of the Ontario Supreme Court is useful:

> "We respect the rights of the individual adult but we tolerate uncontrolled authority over children. We respect the rights of the individual adult while overlooking the constant violation of the rights of children. This paradox is rooted in the age-old relation between a child and his elders. Modern thinking prompts us to ask: Is the child a person with legal rights or merely a body subject to the whims and wishes of whoever may have possession?"[38]

How society deals with child-related law has evolved from four basic historical legal concepts:

- *Patria Potestas (the power of the father)*

- *Parens Patriae* (the state as parent)

- The best interests of the child

- The child as a person before the law.

It is in balancing the four concepts that we as a society address the concerns of children. However, we are not well practiced in thinking of the child as a person before the law with his own interests that need to be accounted for in decision-making. The national task force placed before Canadian society the challenge to see the child as citizen and act accordingly.

Those involved in planning and delivering services to young people need to be aware of their status as citizens with rights. They must go beyond talking about children and planning for them. The title of the report, *Admittance Restricted: The Child as Citizen in Canada* remains an apt description of the current status of young people three decades later. While changes have been made in our approach to children, we still have a ways to go in recognizing their place in society.

THE COMMISSION ON EMOTIONAL AND LEARNING DISORDERS IN CHILDREN (CELDIC)

In 1970 a milestone document was greeted with great public interest. *One Million Children*, produced by the CELDIC committee, was the first national look at the mental health needs of youngsters in Canada.

The Commission was formally established in February 1966 by the following sponsors, representing an impressive array of national organizations:

- The Canadian Association for Retarded Children

- The Canadian Council on Children and Youth

- The Canadian Education Association

- The Canadian Mental Health Association

- The Canadian Rehabilitation Council for the Disabled

- The Canadian Welfare Council

- Dr. Barnardo's of the United Kingdom.

The committee was a broadly based coalition of national voluntary agencies with representatives from all provinces. It was chaired by Charles Roberts from Ontario and Denis Lazure from Quebec both academic psychiatrists responsible for services in university hospital based facilities. The title, *One Million Children* represents the proportion of children deemed by the committee to have special emotional and learning needs based on an incidence of 12 to 15 percent of the population. The Commission created study groups in each province and held meetings across the country. The final report was written on the basis of the provincial meetings. The study groups were made up of professionals from all aspects of services to children and youth.

The introduction of the report focuses the reader on the main theme of the report, the problem of coordination of services:

> "If we were asked to put into a single word what distressed us most we would say *divisions* . . . We divide our services: health, education, welfare, corrections. We provide these through different levels of government, federal, provincial-local and through public and private endeavor. . . . There are many different professions, and they all speak different languages. Their 'tribal jargon' serves to separate the professions from each other and from other potential helpers. No single factor has caused us more concern than the picture of different professions struggling to establish their own power base, distrustful of each other, refusing to share so-called confidential information and in this division frequently failing the child."[39]

This was a central theme in every province – the main problem was that services are poorly coordinated and that the problem of coordinating services needs to be addressed as a first priority. Even in Saskatchewan where there were almost no mental health services for children and youth the professionals focused on coordination of services, not the lack of them.

While a major thrust of the report was to argue for the need for coordinated planning and delivery of services to children the report proceeds to describe the findings by making traditional divisions – separate chapters for each of The Child as Student, Patient, Ward, Offender, in Residential Care. And sadly, the section on the Child as Patient has a very strong focus on hospitals and child psychiatry with many examples from the Ontario and Quebec inpatient units for children and adolescents. Other provinces with lesser populations did not have the capacity to develop services on a child psychiatry based model although a 1964 Report by an interdepartmental committee had recommended that model for Saskatchewan but it was never implemented.[40]

The CELDIC report proposed changes that would redress the balance between central and local decision-making thus encouraging regional or local power, would integrate services and do away with fragmentation and make local community service boards responsible for service delivery. Many decades later many of the problems described by CELDIC remain to plague the service delivery system.

Nevertheless, the overall theme of coordination remained and provided a focus that was to change service delivery for children and youth in Canada in a substantial manner. After CELDIC the systems providing services to children were more aware of the problems that were caused when coordination was not uppermost in planning and delivering services to youngsters.

Problems in coordination of services are still with us thirty-five years later. This is a troublesome issue and the solution eludes the service delivery system. Whenever a group of human service professionals get together to discuss the problems of children, the coordination theme remains a top priority. Even in provinces such as British Columbia with amalgamated services in a single ministry, management structure service coordination remains a problem. There is little doubt that professionals brought together from various agencies and systems are more likely to talk about service delivery than children and youth.

The process that CELDIC undertook was one of "speaking on behalf of children and youth", speaking from the outside, speaking from professional or system stances. However, this broadly based coalition with study committees in each province created the fist national view of services for children and youth, a landmark outcome. The CELDIC Report should be required reading in all professional training schools and by those who plan and deliver services to children and youth.

THE CHILD ABUSE REVOLUTION IN CANADA

In 1962 Henry Kempe and colleagues in Denver Colorado published *The Battered Child Syndrome*.[41] Their analysis drew wide public and professional attention to the complex issues involved in child abuse.

Kempe emphasized the need for a team approach involving health, education, child welfare and the legal systems and the need for long term follow up. Kempe recommended that there be mandatory reporting to the police of all suspected cases of child abuse.

For years the debate continued as to the most appropriate authority to receive reports of cases of abuse – to the civil child welfare authorities or to police as representative of the criminal authority. At the centre of this debate is the question of the approach to be taken – reuniting families or the best interests of the child. The importance of Kempe's work in bringing forward into the public domain the needs of abused children is unquestioned. Kempe, as a physician, caused other physicians, hospitals, and the whole of the health care system to change their approaches and to begin to work in concert with the child welfare and legal systems to address this largely hidden problem.

In Canada, Mary Van Stolk is credited by many as the person who focused the attention of professionals and the public on the problem of child abuse. As founder and president of the Tree Foundation of Canada she worked tirelessly to make known the needs of the battered and abused child and to encourage the development of services to meet those needs.

26

Her 1972 publication, *The Battered Child in Canada*[42] began the revolution that addressed the needs of abused children through changed laws and an interdependent service delivery system focused on the needs of children.

During the 1970s the Government of Canada initiated a number of legislative and advisory committees to make recommendations to provide more effective protection for abused and neglected children. In 1976 the House of Commons Standing Committee on Health, Welfare and Social Affairs made fifteen recommendations based in the statement:

> "Every child should be entitled to adequate protective services in his own home and that these services include support services to parents as well as health and other community services to the child in his own right."[43]

The report called for federal funds to be available for research and assistance to the provinces to establish common information systems, to promote the exchange of information and to create common legislation.

The report recommended amendments to the Criminal Code to allow spouses to give evidence in criminal cases of child abuse. As well, a program of public and professional education was undertaken. Financial support was extended to crisis information services through cost-sharing arrangements with the provinces and in 1978 a federal desk for a Child Abuse Information Program was created and in 1982 incorporated within the mandate of the National Clearinghouse on Family Violence.

Over the next twenty years, the subject of child abuse was the topic of a number of federal and national reports. In 1976 the Advisory Council on the Status of Women made recommendations on changes to the Criminal Code covering offences to children. In 1979, the Law Reform Commission of Canada recommended sweeping changes to the Criminal Code to protect children from abuse. In 1980 the Canadian Commission for the International Year of the Child made recommendations about sexual education, protection from exploitation, pornography and reform of sex crime laws. In 1980 the Standing Committee on Health, Welfare and Science of the Senate published their report *Child at Risk*[43] which focused on early childhood experiences as causes of criminal behaviour.

In 1984 the Badgley Committee summarized the recommendations of the above reports and others in *The Report of the Committee on Sexual Offences Against Children and Youth.*[44] The mandate of the committee was to determine the adequacy of the laws and other means used by the community in providing protection for children and to make recommendations for improving protection. Strengthening the provision of services was seen as a priority to ensure the safety and wellbeing of children. Further, the committee made specific recommendations on juvenile prostitution and child pornography.

The Federal Government response to the Badgley Committee report was swift and included: changes to the Criminal Code and Canada Evidence Act; the establishment of the Family Violence Prevention Division; a $25 million special funding program; and the appointment of a special advisor, Rix Rogers, who was given a mandate to report to the Minister on the development of a long range plan for federal initiatives. Rogers' report, *Reaching for Solutions*[45] followed national consultations that focused on ensuring needs were being addressed across the country. The community development approach taken to gathering data was instrumental in bringing professionals together in each province to identify and resolve problems locally and to provide feedback on proposed national actions.

Since the 1960s the needs of youngsters who are neglected and/or physically and sexually abused have increasingly been met by a service delivery system that has been more effectively working together. The debate continues as to when to protect children by removing them from the family and when to provide family services to keep the child safe and secure within the family. Furthermore, there remains the problem of how to access the resources needed when the abuse takes place outside of the family and consequently the child is not in need of protection. Often the child and family are in need of counseling and other services that may not be readily available outside of the child welfare system. However, those communities that have established a good level of trust in working together are usually able to resolve these issues. Most importantly, sexual offences against children and the protection of children are now in the public domain and children are safer than in the past.

YOUTH HOSTELS AND STREET CLINICS

In the early sixties two intersecting themes converged and, for a short time, attracted a lot of Federal funding. Youth were on the move, traveling across the country and needing places to stay to get them off the street and so municipalities and newly developed community agencies received federal funding to set up a string of youth hostels across the land. And simultaneously, there was rising concern about the illicit use of street drugs and the short term answer was to develop street clinics where youth could receive assistance as needed – those who were traveling and those who were overcome with whatever street drugs were currently available.

Prime Minister Pierre Trudeau led the approach of the federal government to the youth problems of the 1960s. His office employed a group of young men and women as policy advisors to provide the policy and planning advice that formed the basis on which the federal funds were available. By design, both the youth hostel and street clinic movements were youth-involving. Many of those hired to work in the hostels and in the street clinics were youth who might otherwise have been traveling. Youth were recruited to be members of the boards of directors. This peer approach to services provided a new look at how services could be made more sensitive to those in need.

In Regina, the Street Clinic staff endeared themselves to the emergency wards of the hospitals because they began to make themselves available to youth in crisis (often due to illicit drugs). The process of peer involvement and youth empowerment was a new approach to services and an important difference in the way that services were provided. As time went by and federal funds for youth-specific programming dried up, the staff of the Street Clinic in Regina and the programs that were delivered were incorporated into the newly formed Mobile Family Crisis Service. "Mobile" was established to provide after hours and weekend crisis response largely for the child welfare system and in cooperation with the police and the emergency wards.

INTERNATIONAL YEAR OF THE CHILD – 1979

On November 20, 1959 the United Nations General Assembly declared that "Mankind owes the child the best it has to give" and unanimously adopted a resolution setting out the Rights of the Child. On December 21, 1976 this same body adopted a resolution proclaiming 1979 International Year of the Child with the following general objectives:

1. To provide a framework for advocacy on behalf of children and for enhancing the awareness of the special needs of children on the part of decision-makers and the public;

2. To promote recognition of the fact that programs for children should be an integral part of economic and social development plans with a view to achieving in both the long term and short term sustained activities for the benefit of children at the national and international levels.

In September of 1978 the Canadian Commission for the International Year of the Child, with forty-five commissioners from all provinces, was established to promote the widespread involvement of individuals, communities and organizations in activities to advance the rights, interests and well-being of children in the context of families and society. It was not established as a commission of inquiry rather, it followed the lead of the United Nations and stressed promotion and advocacy on behalf of children. It provided an opportunity for those concerned with the welfare of children to come together to share information and plan for a stronger social response to meet their needs. The report of the commission, *For Canada's Children*,[46] reflects what the Commission was told about the status of children in Canada. In the introduction to the report, Landon Pearson now Senator Pearson wrote:

> "As they relate to children, our major economic and cultural structures continue to reflect a mythical period when families were intact, human resources abounded and childhood was a glorious time. The fact that childhood very often was far from carefree did not seem to matter much then. Now we know it does".[47]

The Commission was responsible for a budget of $1 million and received over 4,000 submissions from every part of Canada. Members traveled extensively and met with groups across the country. Recommendations were made in a wide range of areas. The report was focused on prevention by modifying stressful environments and strengthening individual capacities to cope with stress. However, the only recommendation pertinent to mental health was that:

> "The target areas suggested in the family service grid in The State of the Art: A Background Paper on Prevention receive special attention from health professionals and provincial governments".[48]

At the same time the Commission recommended "every province adopt a comprehensive dental-care program for children" and in many other areas of health – best babies, immunization, nutrition, hospitalization, injury prevention, sexuality, health education, fitness and alcohol and drug abuse – they made comprehensive recommendations.

Mental health was not on the radar screen of the Commission in 1979. How could this be so? Well, for one thing, the Canadian Mental Health Association was not a member. The provincial government representatives came from the departments and ministries responsible for child welfare. Within the federal government, leadership for the International Year was established on the welfare side of the National Department of Health and Welfare. In turn they recruited provincial participation through their usual network of provincial child welfare authorities. One can conjecture that no one spoke out loudly enough about children's mental health to be heard.

(For a description of Saskatchewan activities during the International Year of the Child, see Chapter 7).

THE POWER OF PARENTS

From the 1950s onward, parents of children with developmental disabilities were organizing to ensure that their children received needed services in the community. Such parent advocacy groups were a powerful force for change. Parents of children with learning disabilities were instrumental in forcing changes in schools to ensure that their children received appropriate education. In Saskatchewan the Association for Children with Learning Disabilities was a vital agent of change. Parents of children with autism and related disorders organized first in Regina and developed a home-based treatment program funded by the Psychiatric Services Branch. In two provinces, British Columbia and Ontario, parents of children with autism have resorted to the courts to ensure that their children receive appropriate treatment. They have been successful at the federal Supreme Court level in obtaining decisions that require those provinces to provide needed treatment services to assist the development of their children.

YOUTH JUSTICE

Appearing before the Joint Committee of the Senate and of the House of Commons debate on repatriating the constitution of Canada in 1980, David Cruickshank , Joe Ryant and

Andrew Cohen speaking about how the Parliament and the Legislatures protect the rights of children and youth made this statement:

> "Parliament's record is hardly praiseworthy. The Juvenile Delinquent's Act (Canada), hardly changed since 1908,and has been slated for replacement since 1965. Fifteen years after the promises, we are still waiting – and still seeing unacceptable, paternalistic practices carried out under the existing Act".[49]

It was their view that in Canadian law young people do not have the same rights as adults and their special status under the law is unacceptable if you believe that human rights are indivisible and not to be parcelled out to different segments of society under different circumstances. To recognize the individuality of the child's interests before the law is essential in framing a constitution for Canada.

The *Juvenile Delinquents Act (JDA)*[50] of 1908 was a paternalistic mechanism to handle children in conflict with the law. Prior to that statute, no separate treatment of young people occurred within the criminal justice system. "Historically, children were tried alongside adults, upon reaching the age of seven, the common law age of criminal responsibility".[51] The *JDA* is based in the *parens patriae* philosophy – the state standing in place of the parents who were thought to be responsible for the misdemeanours of their children. There was little emphasis on due process in the courts – the right to legal representation and the rules of evidence were relaxed.

The *JDA* was replaced in 1984 by the *Young Offenders Act (YOA)*.[52] The age of criminal responsibility was fixed at twelve. Young offenders were to be made more accountable for their actions and at the same time they were afforded due process protections such as the right to legal representation; the right to consult a parent, lawyer or other person before making a statement; and the right to the least interference with their freedom as was consistent with the protection of society. The *YOA* brings the criminal law in respect of youngsters in line with the *Criminal Code of Canada* that governs criminality for all. One of the main arguments for change was to make the courts tougher – to ensure that youth were held responsible for their criminal acts.

From the point of view of mental health services for youth, the paramount section of the *YOA* is Section 13 which deals with the preparation of reports to the court by physicians, psychiatrists, psychologists and other qualified persons. Under the *JDA* many judges asked for such special reports, however, the *YOA* provides positive encouragement and outlines processes to be used.

The introduction of the *YOA* resulted in the development of specialized forensic mental health services for youth and access to federal monies to establish and maintain such programs. Some jurisdictions, including British Columbia developed a specialized separate program while Saskatchewan incorporated the new services within the Psychiatric Services Branch. The outcome in Saskatchewan has been a much improved service for youth before the law and a closer working relationship between Youth Justice and Mental Health services.

During the next fifteen years there was a reduction in the number of youth court cases. At the same time, the public perception was that youth crime was on the increase. This is an interesting contradiction that has no easy explanation especially when at the same time there was a dramatic increase in the number of youth who were sentenced by the courts to be in custody. The result has been a public call to "get tough" on youth crime.

In 2002 new legislation, the *Youth Criminal Justice Act* (YCJA)[53] was passed and came into force on April 1, 2003. Changes that are important to note include the introduction of the concept of "timeliness" meaning that courts should act quickly to make determinations in respect of young person's perceptions of time between an act and its consequences. As well, the new *Act* requires that the courts "respect gender, ethnic, cultural and linguistic differences and respond to the needs of young aboriginal offenders".

Another section of the *Act* discusses the need to ensure that the actions taken against young offenders should take into account the needs of victims and the community in making decisions. The *YCJA* also increases the importance to be given to front-end or extra-judicial measures that might be taken to hold a young person accountable without appearing in court. There is a new set of sentencing principles that bring the *YCJA* in line with changes to the Criminal Code respecting adult criminality.

There has not been enough experience with the new *YCJA* to be able to compare the results with those of the *YOA*. Time will tell if it is a better approach to youth justice. The same issues remain – getting tough and ensuring accountability versus providing services to ensure that youth grow and develop outside the criminal justice system for the literature shows that incarceration leads to further criminality. It is an ineffective way to prevent crime and protect the public.

The facts about custodial care for youth in Canada are bleak indeed:

> "Adults are incarcerated at a rate of 130 inmates per 100,000 population in Canada, less than the rate in the United States. Yet Canada incarcerates young people under the age of 18 at a much higher rate than adults, 447 per 100,000 population. Moreover, this is considerably higher than the corresponding youth incarceration rate of 311 per 100,000 population in the United States, 86 per 100,000 for Scotland, and 69 per 100,000 population in England and Wales. . . Further, more than one half are incarcerated for property and process offences rather than for offences involving personal injury".[54]

There are elements in the *YCJA* that will make a better system for youth and a difference in the future. These include a new respect for gender, ethnic, and linguistic differences including responding to the needs of Aboriginal youth. A second vital issue within the new Act is the importance of front-end decision-making that will divert youth from the formal court system.

And lastly, removing from the courts the decision about where the youth will be placed whether in open or closed custody and leaving this decision up to the provincial director of youth corrections will be the key to ensuring that these decisions are made in the best interests of youth.

INTERNATIONAL YEAR OF YOUTH (IYY)

In 1985 the United Nations honored youth with an International Year. An important outcome of the year was the increased recognition by society of young people as citizens with individual rights. By determining the age of youth to be aged 15 to 25 for the International Year, teenagers were clustered with young adults for the purposes of social debate. Consequently, issues were raised, debated and decided with new sets of eyes.

At the national level the most important outcome of the year was the establishment of the Canadian Youth Foundation following a legacy grant of one million dollars from the federal government. The Foundation was staffed by youth and the board of directors were predominantly young people under the age of 25. Later the Foundation changed its focus from the analysis of policy from a youth perspective to a program assisting young people to establish small businesses.

In Saskatchewan as in other provinces there was a new focus on the capacity of the young person to consent to health care at age 18 for general health care and 16 for mental health care. The Law Reform Commission of Saskatchewan proposed changes to allow consent for health care to be made by the young person depending upon the youth's capacity to understand the implications of the care to be provided.

Youth participation in society was encouraged by the International Year and important concepts such as peer counselling began to be added to youth-serving programs. While it may seem obvious now to emphasize youth participation – to assert that youth can make a significant contribution to their communities, that they can assume responsible decision-making roles in society – it seemed less obvious prior to the International Year of Youth.

(For a description of a Saskatchewan Health IYY initiative see Chapter 7)

IN CONCLUSION

Many public movements have been instrumental in changing the provision of services to children and youth. In most instances these movements have been centred in federal government priorities and have brought with them federal funds to study issues or provide new sources of funding. Concerns about sexual abuse of children and the need for treatment services and the changes embodied in the Young Offenders Act brought with them new funding to ensure that the mental health needs of these populations were met.

The International Years of the Child (1979) and Youth (1985) provided many opportunities to consider the needs of young people and form new alliances on their behalf or with them.

From the point of view of mental health services for children and youth, the power of parents and other community groups has the most likelihood of making a difference in the future. There has never been a powerful community advocacy group focused on the broader mental health needs of children and youth. It has been demonstrated that organizations of citizens can be very powerful agents for change. The time has come to learn from the lessons of the past and provide the support necessary to bring together those concerned about children and youth and their health.

3

The Mental Hospital Years

IN THE BEGINNING

Saskatchewan was a leader in establishing publicly funded health care in Canada. If we are to understand Canadian health care policy a good place to start is by looking at Saskatchewan's role in its development. The history of the evolution of health care in Saskatchewan, including mental health care, is an important achievement.

From the earliest days there were strong leaders – politicians, professionals and community members with vision, doggedness and skill contributing to the development of social programs in the province.

In the years from the 1880s to the 1960s, Saskatchewan grew from a sparsely settled part of the North West Territories to a well-serviced, well-organized province of almost a million people. The development of mental health services was shaped by a number of factors. There were always the problems caused by a large geography and a widely scattered population. Economic factors beyond the control of the province were critical. The decade of the worldwide economic depression in the 1930s was accompanied by years of drought on the prairies and Saskatchewan was hit particularly hard. Very little was developed during that time and anything that was, was in response to the poverty experienced by almost everyone. Federal decisions with respect to funding have also had an enormous influence in how and what programs develop. And certain individuals, both political and professional played powerful roles in service development.

The growth in health services – particularly mental health services and child health services – in Saskatchewan from the 1880s to the 1960s when the mental hospital era ended and the community psychiatry movement began is worth study. During this time there were no specialized services for children and youth in Saskatchewan and the development of children's services was greatly influenced by the evolution of other health services.

Prior to 1905, legislation governing the North West Territories was enacted by the Government of Canada. Beginning in the 1880s health services were organized under the Department of Agriculture of the Territories. In 1905 when the Province of Saskatchewan was created there were six hospitals operating in the new province and government was subsidizing hospital care at the rate of ten cents per patient per day plus fifty cents per day for indigent patients.

By 1915 there were 28 hospitals in settled parts of the province. In 1920 the Red Cross Society began operating outpost hospitals in remote areas. During the depression in the 1930s hospital construction was halted but it was resumed again as a major focus of development during the years after World War Two.

Saskatchewan people are very proud of the significant role that the cooperative movement has played in the development of the province. People learned early the value of working together. Johnson describes this well in *Dream No Little Dreams*.

> "The settler felt alone; alone against the elements, alone in his efforts to develop his farm, alone against the organizations that supplied his needs and bought his products,

and alone even against those who governed him from Ottawa. Here was fertile ground for co-operation and community action."[55]

The Saskatchewan Wheat Pool organized by farmers so they could market their grain together was an early example of a pattern of cooperative endeavours that has continued throughout the history of the province. In the 1920s rural municipal governments developed an indigenous system of socialized medicine with doctors on salary and union hospitals.

The first mental health legislation in what is now Saskatchewan was the *Safe Keeping of Dangerous Lunatics in the North West Territories Act of 1879* which provided for the removal of insane persons to the Stony Mountain Penitentiary in Manitoba. In 1885 legislation[56] was passed to provide the authority to transfer insane persons from the Manitoba penitentiary to the Selkirk Lunatic Asylum or any other provincial asylum. Compensation was made to the government of Manitoba for the care and maintenance of insane persons. The Brandon Institution was converted in 1891 to an asylum to serve western Canada, the North West Territories and the Yukon. When a person was deemed to be insane institutional or asylum care was the usual response.

Institutional care had a cost and there was a clear expectation that this cost would be paid by the individual or family members. In 1906, the Province of Saskatchewan passed the *Insanity Act*.

Chapter 22 Section 6 stated: "If the Justice is satisfied that the person so apprehended as aforesaid is insane and dangerous to be at large it shall also be the duty of said justice to make inquiry whether such person is possessed of any and what property." And further in Section 15: "all expenses incurred in connection with the apprehension, examination, committal to gaol and maintenance of said person unless the same has been otherwise provided by relatives or friends shall be borne by the said insane person." And further, "the government of Saskatchewan shall be entitled to recover the said expenses from and out of the estate of the said insane person or from the persons found to be legally liable to provide for this care and maintenance." And in Section 17, "When an indigent person is committed to an asylum and is not possessed of sufficient means or the relatives of such person are incapable of providing the same, the cost of his maintenance and other expenses shall be defrayed by the province."[57]

From the initial establishment of the province, the province paid for institutional care only for those who could not do so and the government of the day showed a keen concern with costs. As with other forms of health care at this time, the individual or the family was responsible for the costs of mental health care.

In 1906 Saskatchewan began to plan the first mental hospital and a Memorandum re: Asylum from the Department of Public Works tells part of the story:

> "There seems to be no model building in Manitoba to get ideas from, the Brandon Asylum having been an old building remodelled and added to at several different times. . . . We should acquire at least a half section of land to be worked in connection with the asylum and by the patients, it being admitted that such diversion is essential to the majority of such cases. The province of Manitoba is running their asylum farms to a profit. We find that 'work' is a useful diversion for the mentally ill and the asylum farm provides a useful form of income to the province."[58]

Again, the concern for money to pay for care is an issue of importance and the type of care that was planned appeared to include work which would be therapeutic.

The *Insanity Act of 1906* included mention of Saskatchewan's aboriginal people. The financial policy "Re: Indians" was clear. "Indians shall not be removed to a hospital unless the cost of their maintenance and other charges are guaranteed by the Superintendent General of Indian Affairs."[59] The federal government was to pay for their care.

In 1907 a report was prepared by Dr. David Low that might be considered the first Saskatchewan Plan for Psychiatric Services.[60] Low was physician to Premier Walter Scott and his report led to the construction of the Battleford Mental Hospital. The relationship between Scott and Low is important as it reveals one of the most important factors in understanding government decision-making. In making change governments often act slowly, however, when a senior politician forms a partnership with a knowledgeable and trusted professional change can happen much more quickly.

In part, the Low report states "the modern idea is to remove all evidence of restraint in the management of the insane." And further, "instead of measures of restraint such as padded cells and strait jackets they are allowed their freedom, sufficient attendants being supplied to take proper care of them." And further "soothing remedies are employed as baths and sedative medicines."

Low also provides a full description of the type of facility he proposes.

> "Stress on the necessity of securing an abundance of land . . . of the very best and richest of farming land. Employment in the open air has been found one of the most efficient methods of bringing about recovery . . . various employments of agriculture constitute the most easily provided means of supplying this essential in the pleasantest and most acceptable way to the patients."

Low's report provided a thoughtful compilation of the then available best practices in psychiatric care.

In 1912, a Petition to the Provincial Executive Council led to the appointment of the first superintendent of the Battleford institution. "We the undersigned members of the Legislative Assembly respectfully suggest that Dr. MacNeill of Hanley be appointed superintendent of the hospital for the insane at Battleford.[61] For over thirty years Dr. J. W. MacNeill was the undoubted leader of the provincial program. He remained in charge at North Battleford until 1945 and in his later years he provided provincial leadership as first Commissioner of Mental Health.

In 1913 the Saskatchewan Hospital at North Battleford was opened with the following admissions policy – all patients were committed on orders by provincial magistrates. The Department of Public Works was responsible for the mental hospital program. The rationale for this was probably because the hospital was housed in a series of government buildings that needed to be maintained. In the winter of 1914 a total of 346 Saskatchewan residents who were patients in the Brandon Asylum were transferred by train to the Battleford hospital. The institution grew quickly and by April 30, 1915, housed 501 patients.

In 1914 an *Act to Appoint an Administrator of Lunatics' Estates* was proclaimed. It gave the administrator guardianship of the estates of those detained in public asylums with the

> "power and authority ... to mortgage or sell such real estate or any portion thereof and to execute the necessary transfers . . . (when) profits and income of the real estate are insufficient for the maintenance of the lunatic or his family or for the education of his children, or that it is desirable in the interests of the lunatic and his estate that the property should be sold or mortgaged."[62]

For many years to come the province was to be concerned about the costs of mental health care and how it was to be financed.

In the 1916 Annual Report of the Department of Public Works MacNeill noted increases in admissions.

> "I have to report a steady increase in our population, especially is this true from the rural districts . . . it is painful to see the large number coming suffering from different forms of mental depression and mental confusion due to isolation. We have also a number of those women who break down nervously after confinement."[63]

And in his next Annual Report to the Department of Public Works MacNeill wrote:

> "I receive many letters . . . where a patient whose mental condition needs treatment and who would be willing to have treatment if he were being sent to any place but the asylum or the hospital for the insane as this place is called. I would respectfully ask that the title of the Insanity Act be changed so that all reference to 'Insanity' be eliminated."[64]

What we now term politically correct language was a concern then and the power of labels was acknowledged. Terms such as lunacy and mental degenerate were disturbing and did not encourage public understanding or acceptance of treatment.

In 1917 Gerhard Ens, MLA, for Rosthern wrote an inspector's report to the Department of Public Works. He stated that "The farm needs more horses and cattle. If more horses could be bought for the institution, a great deal more land could be brought under cultivation, which to my mind would help a great deal towards the up keep."[65] Meaningful work and income for the hospital remained an issue of concern to the government.

The North Battleford Hospital was becoming overcrowded and in 1921, Weyburn Hospital was opened. In his first Annual Report, Dr. W. A. Mitchell observed " . . . we have only been open for patients for four and a half months. However, in that time we have admitted 607 patients; of these 114 are new admissions and 493 transfers from Battleford, Brandon, Regina and Wolseley."[66] The transfers from Regina and Wolseley came from the local hospitals and care facilities for the elderly.

Politically correct language arises again in 1922 when new legislation is passed to change the name to the *Administrator of Estates of the Mentally Incompetent* from the former *Administrator of Lunatic's Estates.*[67]

The first written evidence of the medicalization of

mental health services in Saskatchewan occurred in 1922 when MacNeill wrote in his eighth North Battleford Hospital Annual Report, "I am pleased to note that the legislation (the new *Mental Diseases Act*) takes into account that a disease process is being dealt with, rather than a criminal prosecution." The government, through its legislation, now recognized the process of mental disease rather than a personal status of lunacy requiring custodial care. This is particularly significant because disease processes can be treated.[68]

Mitchell's second Weyburn Hospital Annual Report of 1923 discusses an expansion of services.

> "School for Defectives: We got this department opened last September . . . We have 180 defectives but of those 151 are either idiots or imbeciles, and can be taught practically nothing."[69]

Almost thirty years later in 1952, those concerned with services for people with developmental disabilities, primarily their parents, pressured the government until a specialized program for people who were deemed mentally retarded was developed at the Training School (now Valley View Centre) in Moose Jaw. In the next twenty years the term mental defective was replaced by the term mentally retarded and later by developmentally delayed.

MacNeill's tenth Annual Report in 1924 describes the situation in Battleford and makes a plea for improvements:

> "Insufficient staff and especially insufficient medical staff . . . it is 'penny wise and pound foolish'. The place of detention must give way to the hospital, and to the up-to-date, well-equipped hospital, if the state is going to be relieved of the economic burden imposed upon it, even a degree."[70]

Throughout the years MacNeill's annual reports described the changes that he deemed necessary to provide better services. However, as noted before, the committed and knowledgeable professional is insufficient to cause dramatic change. Professional commitment must be matched with political commitment for change to proceed. It took many years for Saskatchewan to act upon MacNeill's dream of "the up-to-date, well-equipped hospital."

THE DEPARTMENT OF HEALTH IS ESTABLISHED IN 1923

The Public Health Act of 1909 created a Bureau of Health that remained a part of the Department of Agriculture until 1923 when the Department of Health was established. However, until 1944, mental health services remained in the administration of the Department of Public Works whose main responsibility was to administer government buildings. The two mental hospitals were two of the largest government buildings in the province and employed the greatest number of staff.

Before 1909 public health services included the collection of vital statistics plus bacteriology and laboratory facilities. The priority was concerns about epidemic disease. The new Bureau of Health introduced preventive programs to ensure the safety of water supplies, sewage disposal and milk distribution. The Bureau began school and public health nursing services and established free communicable disease control service. In 1916 up-to-date health promotion was encouraged by the purchase of a moving picture projector and films dealing with venereal disease, tuberculosis, milk and baby welfare.[71]

In 1916, Saskatchewan enacted the first municipal doctor legislation in North America. *The Municipal Hospital Act* permitted rural municipalities to supplement the income of physicians by way of a grant of up to $1500 per year. Further, in 1919 new legislation allowed municipalities to hire physicians on a salary not to exceed $5,000 per year to provide free medical care to residents. By 1927 there were 13 municipal doctors working in rural municipalities and the number increased to 32 physicians in 1930 and to 173 in 1950. A salary encouraged physicians to establish rural practices during the depression years when money was scarce. The system was important to doctors and especially valuable to people living in rural areas.

The *Municipal Hospital Act* also allowed rural municipalities to work together to erect and maintain hospitals. Union Hospital Districts were quickly established – ten in 1920 and twenty by 1930. However, the depression years brought poverty and little new union hospital development.

Following the election of the CCF government and the Sigerest Report of 1944 there was a new emphasis on union hospitals. By 1947, the seventy-eight UHDs

> "covered more than one-third of the settled area of the province, included approximately one-third of the population and provided three-eighths of the hospital beds.[72]

In 1924 the Junior Red Cross opened the first children's hospital in Regina. During World War I Junior Red Cross Clubs were organized in classrooms across the province and students collected money to assist needy crippled children and as well to provide traveling medical and dental clinics throughout the province. In 1949 the small children's hospital moved to the Regina General Hospital and provided services for crippled children until 1962 when the hospital took over management responsibility for the paediatric ward component and the rehabilitation functions were transferred to Wascana Hospital.

Primarily due to periodic polio epidemics, rehabilitation units were established in Saskatoon in 1943 and in Regina in 1947. The units also provided treatment for those with cerebral palsy and other chronic disabling conditions. In 1950 a group of Saskatoon parents of children with cerebral palsy established a new voluntary organization, the Saskatchewan Council for Crippled Children and Adults, later the Saskatchewan Abilities Council. The Council operated traveling clinics throughout the province from the early fifties through the 1960s and was responsible for establishing the Children's Rehabilitation Centre. With the development of the Saskatchewan Council for Crippled Children and Adults we see in Saskatchewan a third force to create change in health care – the development of a coalition of interested citizens to provide pressure for change. Citizen pressure groups have been instrumental in supporting committed professionals to effect change and have been even more successful in convincing politicians that change is needed.

In 1925, Dr. F.C. Middleton, the first Deputy Minister of Health, in his annual report to the Saskatchewan Government, quoted the President of the American Child Public Health Association on the question of child's Bill Of Rights:

> "There should be no child:
> * That has not been born under proper conditions
> * That does not live in hygienic surroundings
> * That suffers from under-nutrition
> * That does not have prompt and efficient medical attention and inspection
> * That does not receive primary instruction in the elements of hygiene and good health."[73]

Middleton and the American Public Health Association did not mention a child's mental health needs. One hopes that more than seventy-five years later that the living standards of Saskatchewan's children have exceeded those laid down by Middleton and especially that their mental health needs are being met.

In 1921 the first sanatorium for the treatment of tuberculosis was opened and in 1929 Saskatchewan legislated free care for tuberculosis – a first for Canada. The costs of treatment were to be met by levies on urban and rural governments and supplemented by per diem grants from the province.

1930 was an important year for the development of mental health services in Saskatchewan. Dr. C.M. Hincks of the National Committee for Mental Hygiene delivered a report to the government *"Provincial Mental Hospitals and Mental Hygiene Conditions in the Province of Saskatchewan"*.[74] The report commented on overcrowding in both Weyburn and Battleford hospitals, deplored that there was no formal training for personnel and recommended that mental defectives be removed from Weyburn Hospital to a suitably constructed institution.

In 1931 Saskatchewan established its first non-institutional mental health facility at Regina General Hospital – the Psychopathic Ward. This was followed by the establishment of the first traveling community clinic in 1939.

In 1936 new legislation – the *Mental Hygiene Act* included, for the first time, a provision for voluntary admission for inpatient care and gave physicians the authority to certify that patients needed inpatient care in addition to the magistrates' committal which previously had been the only entry to inpatient care.

In 1937, Dr C. Hincks of the National Committee for Mental Hygiene wrote another report to Cabinet. In a letter to the Minister of Health, Dr. J.M. Uhrich, Hincks notes that Saskatchewan Hospital North Battleford designed for 900 now has 1,391 patients and Saskatchewan Hospital Weyburn designed for 1,350 now has 1,790. "All in all arrangements would be considered inadequate for animals." He recommended a new hospital be built at Saskatoon for an immediate population of 1,500 with eventual capacity for 2,000.[75]

As this phase of Saskatchewan's history, the first forty years, closes it is important to note that while many advances had taken place in health care including mental health care the predominant model remained custodial care in mental hospitals. There were still no mental health services for children and youth and no development plans in place. Early planning for rural municipalities to construct and operate hospitals was slowed by the depression years but the successful model was in place and working well where it existed. The Municipal Doctor Plan maintained primary health care services in the rural areas throughout the province during the depression. The depression and war years were not years of growth and development in health care or any human service.

THE CCF YEARS – 1944 TO 1964

A new era in health care in Saskatchewan began following the election of the Co-operative Commonwealth Federation or CCF the first successful socialist government in North America. The CCF was committed to economic and social security for everyone. Probably the most important aspect to social security was hospital and medical care. Their program included

> "the establishment of a complete system of socialized health services so that all would receive adequate medical, surgical, dental, nursing and hospital care without charge."[76]

From the time he became Premier in 1944 until 1949 Premier T.C. Douglas took the unusual step of taking responsibility for the Department of Public Health. He could not have found a better way to communicate clearly how important he thought this was and he was a powerful and effective leader for change in health care. By keeping the health portfolio in the premier's office he ensured that health care was the government priority. Through his leadership in Saskatchewan Douglas was one of the architects of Canada's health care system.

One of the first major undertakings of the new government was to establish the Saskatchewan Health Services Survey – a Royal Commission conducted by Dr. Henry Sigerist from Johns Hopkins University. Within one month of its appointment, the Commission submitted a broad range of recommendations and equally quickly, the government responded and promised to 'fulfill the spirit of this report' as soon as possible. The recommendations formed the basis of the health system that was built over the CCF's term in office beginning with a structure for public health (including health regions, technical assistance for the development of sewer and water services, mental health clinics, dental clinics), a system for medical and hospital services (including district and tertiary services) and the Commission recommended an array of free services (treatment in mental hospitals and clinics, cancer treatment and treatment of venereal disease).[77] The basic structure would later be the foundation for a universal government-operated hospital insurance plan.

In 1947 Saskatchewan established a comprehensive, publicly financed hospital insurance program – a first in Canada and the model that was to be implemented across the country in years to come.

In 1942-43 the Office of the Administrator of Estates collected $725,000 which represented one third of the expenditure for all medical and non-medical salaries at the two mental hospitals in North Battleford and Weyburn. However, one of Sigerist's most important recommendations was that charges to mental patients and their relatives be discontinued.

A Liberty magazine article, February 8, 1947, *"Canada's Shame: Our Mental Hospitals"* noted:

> "Since 1945, the mental hospitals have been free to all citizens of Saskatchewan of 12 months standing – a step forward. Every other province in Canada still charges all patients who can pay."[78]

At the same time, the new government commissioned the ubiquitous Dr. Clarence Hincks of the National Committee for Mental Health to do his third Saskatchewan survey exclusively concerned with the psychiatric system.

The Hincks Survey of 1945 reported that the two mental hospitals had a combined population of 4,201 with adequate accommodations for only 2,214. He echoed earlier reports that he had made to the government of Saskatchewan:

- Separation of services for the mentally ill, the retarded and epileptics

- Transfer of responsibility for operations to the Department of Public Health

- Establishment of mental hygiene clinics in association with general hospitals in Saskatoon and Regina and staffed with psychiatrists, psychologists, social workers and nurses, and traveling clinics to eight other centres.

- The ultimate aim is to have psychiatric services in all general hospitals and thus eliminate the stigma of the mental hospitals.[79]

Dickinson summarizes the impact of the two reports:

> "Sigerist and Hincks both outlined comprehensive plans for the transformation of psychiatric work and the transition to community psychiatry in Saskatchewan." [80]

MacNeill retired as Commissioner of Mental Health Services in 1945 and Dr D. G. McKerracher was appointed Commissioner in 1946. With the support of Premier Douglas he led the process to change the system of care for the mentally ill. McKerracher was another leader who had an enormous influence on the development of mental health services in Saskatchewan.[81] Although his focus was on services for adults, some of the initiative that he introduced helped pave the way for the later development of mental health services for children. This would include the development of permanent outpatient clinics and engaging the public in mental health issues.

At this time, the total mental hospital patient population was over 4,200. With the move of 700 mental defectives to the former RCAF airport in Weyburn 300 of the most difficult to manage mental defectives remained in the mental hospital in Weyburn.

In 1947 McKerracher introduced a 500 hour training program in psychiatric nursing replacing the staff training program that had been in place since 1931. This was the first psychiatric nursing program to be developed in North America[82] and was a bold and far-sighted move by McKerracher which made possible the eventual role of psychiatric nurses in Saskatchewan's community psychiatry programs. At the same time, over 100 public health nurses received one month orientation training to prepare them to provide community services and follow up care for discharged mental patients.

The Sigerist Commission had recommended the establishment of mental health clinics as part of the health region organization under the direction of regional medical officers of health and the *Mental Hygiene Act* established a new form of care – mental hygiene clinics. Under McKerracher's leadership, in 1947, the first psychiatric out-patient clinic was established at the Munroe Wing of Regina General Hospital with a part time psychiatrist, a psychologist and a social worker. While it was located on the grounds of the General Hospital, Munroe Wing and Clinic were administered directly by government in an arrangement similar to that of the mental hospitals. Saskatoon opened an out patient clinic in 1949 at MacNeill Clinic. Part time clinics opened in Moose Jaw in 1948 followed by clinics in Yorkton, Swift Current, Weyburn, Assiniboia, North Battleford and Prince Albert in the next two years.

In 1950, in order to manage a changing system the Division of Mental Health Services was reorganized into the Psychiatric Services Branch of the Department of Public Health with McKerracher as the director of the provincial program. Prior to this time the two hospitals acted independently with separate hiring and personnel policies. With the establishment of the Psychiatric Services Branch, hiring was centralized into the headquarters and initiatives introduced to ensure that the hospitals had standard personnel and clinical practices.

In 1950 construction began for a new training school for mental defectives in Moose Jaw. It opened in 1952 with the transfer of 1200 patients from the Weyburn hospital to the new institution. In 1962 a former tuberculosis sanatorium in Prince Albert was converted to a second institution for the mentally retarded. At this same time, in response to criticisms by the Saskatchewan Association for Retarded Children, community services were being developed and large numbers of younger and more able patients were discharged to community services and began to receive services in their home communities instead of being institutionalized.

In 1955 McKerracher left the Psychiatric Services Branch to become head of psychiatry at University Hospital in Saskatoon and was replaced as director by Dr. F.S. Lawson who remained until 1965. Lawson was a prominent community psychiatrist whose name is often associated with the Saskatchewan Plan for Mental Health Services – a means for providing psychiatric services to a dispersed rural population. [83]

McKerracher, Humphrey Osmond, the director of the mental hospital in Weyburn and Lawson had conceived the plan and it was then developed by Lawson. The plan recommended that, as a way of dealing with the overcrowding in Battleford and Weyburn, services should be provided closer to home through regional centres. At this time, the Department of Health operated the two large mental hospitals in Weyburn and Battleford serving the south and north of the province and providing long-term treatment and custodial services. Psychiatric wards attached to general hospitals in Regina, Saskatoon and Moose Jaw provided short-term inpatient care and referred patients to the mental hospitals if longer term care was required. The two mental hospitals were overcrowded and understaffed. Patients had limited contact with treatment staff and there was a lack of individualized treatment or rehabilitation planning. Patient care was criticized as being overly regimented, dehumanizing and primarily custodial in nature. This had been noted by Hincks in his three reports to the government.

The central feature of Lawson's plan was to divide the province into regions with approximately equal populations and to administer mental health services locally from these regional centres thus focusing on community mental health services rather than depending upon institutions. The plan proposed that regional mental hospitals be built in Regina, Saskatoon, Yorkton, Prince Albert and three other cities. The facilities at Weyburn and Battleford were to be downsized and the new units were to range in size from 148 to 418 beds. They would be built adjacent to or integrated with existing hospitals. Outpatient departments would be established to provide follow up care. Services such as day programs, night admissions, hostel accommodation and weekend treatment were to be developed.

The Lawson Plan was never fully implemented. It was costly and when in August of 1958 the Federal government announced that they would not cost share such psychiatric institutions the Lawson plan was doomed. The Federal government opted instead to cost share psychiatric units in general hospitals to provide active treatment in the acute phases of mental illness. The specific exclusion of mental hospitals from cost-sharing marked the demise of Lawson's original plan. Decisions about funding almost always drive program development. At the same time, psychotropic drugs were being introduced. They gave psychiatrists and general practitioners effective new ways to treat mental illness and keep people out of hospital or decrease the length of time spent in hospital. Demand for long-term psychiatric beds began to decrease dramatically.

The 1950s and 1960s were heady days for adult psychiatry in Saskatchewan. Interesting research was underway on the biochemical basis of schizophrenia by Dr. Abram Hoffer in Saskatoon. While his theories eventually fell into disrepute, his research attracted considerable attention and substantial research funding. It was believed at the time that lysergic acid diethylamine -25 (LSD) might aid in the understanding of the neurochemical origins of schizophrenia and there was considerable research into using LSD in therapy. General research into the psychology and sociology of mental illness was also underway, particularly in Weyburn and this included early work on the exploration of public attitudes towards mental illness.[84]

During the 1950s and 1960s community resources were being developed and public attitudes were changing. For some years Lawson and McKerracher continued to argue for and support the development of small mental hospitals. Eventually McKerracher undertook a series of studies to determine if psychiatric care in general hospitals with psychiatric consultation, trained staff and psychotropic drugs would be a useful form of care and found this to be so. On the basis of this research he began to advocate that all psychiatric patients be treated in general hospital wards by general practitioners with psychiatric consultants available. He maintained that even specialized psychiatric wards were unnecessary. The pilot projects demonstrated that primary care physicians could manage patients who were mentally ill when psychiatric consultation was available. However, in the final analysis, physician turnover in small communities and the geography of Saskatchewan which limited psychiatric consultation, made it impossible to implement his plan province-wide.

Along with the committed professional leadership of McKerracher and then Lawson, there was considerable popular community support for the Saskatchewan Plan as the embodiment of humane care for the mentally ill. The Canadian Mental Health Association, Saskatchewan Division was the main force that ensured that this support remained strong. The CMHA at this time was an active and articulate advocate for the improvement of mental health services. CMHA (Sask) had strong links with the government (Douglas and all his cabinet were members) and with the Psychiatric Services Branch (all of the senior psychiatrists were members).[85] Even the provincial Liberal Party, in opposition at the time, became vocal supporters of the plan because of the advocacy of the Canadian Mental Health Association.

In 1960, as part of the CCF election platform, construction of a 148 bed mental hospital in Yorkton was announced. However, construction did not start until 1963 and the facility was opened in October of that year. The Yorkton Psychiatric Centre was built on the grounds of the Union Hospital and provided the model for community mental health services in Saskatchewan. It should be noted that the total number of beds constructed (1.8 beds per thousand population) was a considerable decrease from the original plan (5 beds per thousand population). The facility has never been used as a community mental hospital providing long-term care. It has always been an acute care facility with an average length of stay well below thirty days.

At the same time, between 1961 and 1966 a variation on the Saskatchewan Plan was developed and began to be implemented. Saskatchewan Plan 2 was focused on deinstitutionalization and community psychiatry. The goal of deinstitutionalization was to eliminate the large mental hospitals by discharging the patients into community care provided by the regional psychiatric centres. The concept of community psychiatry had other wider goals that included:

- developing community services which would reduce the need for long term inpatient care;

- extending treatment services to persons in the community who had a mental illness but did not require inpatient care; and

- developing services that would prevent mental illness from occurring.

Between 1961 and 1966, deinstitutionalization took place quickly at the mental hospital in Weyburn under the leadership of Dr. Frederic Grunberg and Dr. Hugh Lafave. The patient count dropped from 1,478 to 501. This is the largest decrease in mental hospital patients in the shortest period of time ever in North America.[86] In 1974 the Weyburn facility was transformed into a long-term nursing care facility for the remaining 300 elderly patients. This change of designation was facilitated by new Federal/Provincial funding agreements whereby facilities for the chronically ill elderly were to be cost shared. By 1981, the Battleford hospital had only 250 long term patients remaining and plans were in place to develop a long-term care nursing facility.

By the end of the 1960s, there were eight psychiatric

service regions in the province and each was responsible for services in a defined catchment area. Rather than building small mental hospitals, each region developed an inpatient unit attached to the local hospital and an outpatient program to provide community follow up to those who had been discharged and outpatient services to those who did not need to be admitted. Regional boarding homes known as approved homes were developed for those with chronic conditions. With these changes, by 1981, the average length of inpatient stay across the province was reduced to 23 days and of the 13,500 patients who received services, over 60% received only outpatient care.

Two factors are important to consider when evaluating the changes to mental health services in Saskatchewan in the 1960s. First, the development of psychotropic drugs greatly reduce the need for long-term inpatient care for many disorders. Secondly, in 1968 the joint Federal-Provincial funded health insurance plan was created and funded psychiatric treatment in hospitals and by physicians rather than funding "mental hospital care". This reduced the province's costs for developing and managing the new system of care. While the original Saskatchewan Plan of small regional mental hospitals was never fully implemented, nevertheless, Saskatchewan led the way in Canada by linking a very active deinstitutionalization with the development of community mental health services.

The revolution that took place in Saskatchewan in psychiatric care has provided the model for Canada and much of the United States. The ongoing leadership of Douglas as Premier and the professional expertise of McKerracher and Lawson provided the focus, expertise and enthusiasm to make it work. The strong support of the community through the CMHA ensured that the issue remained high on the politcians' list of priorities. It is largely due to the CMHA involvement that the opposition Liberal Party made the plan one of their election platform planks. Thus with the change of government in 1964 Ross Thatcher and the Liberals who replaced the NDP were committed to the plan's continuation.

However, the plan was focused on providing community services on behalf of adults with mental illness. There was no parallel enthusiasm in the professional or political leadership to develop services for children and youth nor was there a community of concern in the CMHA or any other organization to advocate on behalf of mental health services for youngsters.

4

Setting the Stage

IN THE BEGINNING

By the beginning of the 1950s the principles that would later underpin the development of child and youth programs in Saskatchewan were evolving.

There had been growing demand for mental health services for children and youth and some services were being offered in communities where there was professional staff with an interest in providing such services. There was now a new category of employee in the provincial public service – the educational psychologist – and the eventual home of this new professional helped shape children's services in the province. A number of national and provincial reports were published during this period describing the need for more services for children and youth culminating in the most important of these – the 1970 CELDIC Report, *One Million Children. (see Chapter 2)*

In the early 1960s the Royal University Hospital in Saskatoon established a program of specialized child psychiatry services in which child psychiatrists with joint appointments in the College of Medicine at the University of Saskatchewan, provided out-patient assessment, treatment and consultation services to children from across the province. The service delivery model included social workers, psychologists and other ancillary staff to support medical specialists and residents. This was a unique service in the province and played a very important role in providing assessments for special needs including designations for funding under the Education Act. Six beds for children and youth were designated on the inpatient unit in the 1970s and were the only specialized beds for this population in Saskatchewan until the Adolescent Mental Health Unit was established at Regina General Hospital in 2004.

In 1970 the outpatient program moved from the hospital to Ellis Hall on the university campus. An off-campus out-patient program and a specialized group home, both intended for youth over 12 years, were successfully developed in the following decade. With the creation of the Saskatoon Health District Board in the 1990s the University Hospital and MacNeill Clinic programs were amalgamated.

During the 1950s and 1960s, the outpatient community mental health clinics in Regina, Saskatoon at MacNeill Clinic and University Hospital and Moose Jaw along with associated traveling clinics began to accept referrals of children and youth. There were also small outpatient clinics attached to the mental hospitals in Weyburn and North Battleford.

While there was no staff specifically hired or trained to provide services to youngsters, existing staff gradually expanded their mandate to include young people. In 1967 the MacNeill Clinic in Saskatoon became a designated service for children and in 1968 a second specialized clinic focused on children and families was established in Regina.

It is interesting to note that as early as 1952 with demand outstripping capacity in the community mental health clinics, it was recognized that children and youth ought to be a priority for the new community mental health facilities. "The needs of such groups are great and rewards highest in terms of the most economical use of the facilities available and the return to society."[87]. This argument for a prevention/early intervention approach was never put into practice mainly because of the pressure to discharge adults from the institutions and because of the lack of trained manpower.[88]

A further factor limiting development was the lack of any leadership within the Government or the Psychiatric Services Branch to ensure an early intervention approach serving children and youth. Lastly, there was no organized concerted public effort pressuring the government to provide mental health services to children and youth.

EDUCATIONAL PSYCHOLOGY

The fact of mental disorder in children and the need not just for acute care but for early intervention and preventive services were first presented to the provincial government by S.R. Laycock in the *Commissioner's Report on Mental Hygiene Conditions*. Laycock stated:

> "[I]n the absence of preventive measures more than four per cent of all school children in Saskatchewan will sooner or later become victims of mental illness requiring treatment in a psychiatric setting . . . more than two per cent of children in school attendance are so retarded mentally that they could not profit by regular school curriculum." [89]

Laycock, who was professor of educational psychology at the University of Saskatchewan, went on to develop school psychology services.

Much of the information in this section on educational psychology in Saskatchewan is from a paper by Dave Treherne who was the provincial consultant for this program in the 1970s.[90]

Laycock was employed by the Saskatoon School Board in 1929 and was Saskatchewan's first educational psychologist. For most of his career, he was a professor in the College of Education at the University of Saskatchewan and was a community leader and a noted public advocate for mental health. He was a pioneer in promoting good home-school communication and was the first president of the Saskatchewan

Home and School Association from 1938-42. In 1950 the Canadian National Committee on Mental Hygiene became the Canadian Mental Health Association and the CMHA set up a pilot project in Saskatchewan. Laycock was asked to organize the new Saskatchewan Division and he became the founding president.

In 1947, Laycock along with J.D.M. Griffin, Director of the CMHA and W. Line of the University of Toronto, developed a program "to train selected teachers to work in a liaison capacity between the home and the school in order to promote the best possible milieu through which children's mental health could be fostered." This was a follow up to *The Manual for Teachers: Mental Hygiene* published in 1940 by the trio – Griffin, Laycock and Line.[91]

In 1947, with the support of the Federal Government's Dominion-Provincial Health Grants, Saskatchewan, along with other provinces, developed a new class of employee, the educational psychologist, to provide mental health consultation services for children in schools. The new program was initially administered by the Psychiatric Services Branch with the employees seconded to work under the supervision of the school superintendents. By 1964 the employees had been transferred to the newly established Public Health Regions where the educational psychologists worked alongside the public health nurses providing liaison services between schools and homes. This change of administration for the educational psychologists provided them with a home base in a setting removed from the stigma of mental illness but distanced them from the other mental health disciplines in the Psychiatric Services Branch. One can only speculate that a mental health service for children and youth might have developed earlier had the educational psychologists remained with the other mental health professionals. The program was staffed by teachers who had received bursaries from the province to attend the University of Toronto's Institute of Child Study to earn diplomas in child development. The training program continued until 1970 by which time universities across the country had established graduate degrees in educational psychology.

By 1979 there were 14 educational psychologists serving a total population of 650,000 in the ten rural health regions. Regina and Saskatoon were not covered by this initiative because the public health departments in the two cities were operated by the municipalities and their school boards had developed educational psychology services within their organizations.

The educational psychologists worked with the public health nurses, speech therapists and audiologists providing services to youngsters. Screening activities in the schools and public health preschool clinics provided an ongoing source of youngsters in need of assessment and consultative guidance from educational psychologists. The educational psychologists worked closely with schools and teachers to provide consultation advice on behalf of troubled youngsters. A personal communication with Mary Jean Martin, one of the early educational psychologists, indicates that there was little contact between the pubic health staff and the Psychiatric Services Branch staff in the regions during the 1950s and 1960s.

In the early 1970s the Federal-Provincial Cost-sharing agreements were changed and educational psychologists were no longer eligible for 75% cost-sharing. The population was too small, the distances too great and the program too weak to withstand the loss of federal funding. Too little meaningful contact had been developed within the Ministry of Health between the educational psychologists and the developing Child and Youth Mental Health Service in the Psychiatric Services Branch. There had been little support within the Community Health Services Branch for an amalgamation of health services for children under their auspices following the Review of Child and Youth Health Services in 1979. *(See Chapter 5 for a complete description).*

As a result of the loss of cost-sharing, ten of the educational psychologists were transferred to regional offices in the Department of Education to provide assessments geared to determining levels of disability for the purposes of high and low cost funding and to support the developing special education initiatives of the Department of Education. The model used to fund these positions was a shared services model developed so that smaller school boards could participate in a shared services agreement and thus receive specialist services from a pool of professionals employed by the Department. The major job of the educational psychologists became one of screening and testing to determine if children met the requirements for special education funding from the Department of Education.

The Department of Health was left with four staff now called early childhood psychologists for 10 community health regions, no strategy for serving Regina and Saskatoon, no clear program guidelines or direction and no mechanism for integrating these services with other child health services

1964 – THE FIRST SASKATCHEWAN STUDY OF EMOTIONALLY DISTURBED CHILDREN

In 1963 the Interdepartmental Coordinating Committee on Rehabilitation struck a subcommittee on services to emotionally disturbed children in Saskatchewan. Their findings were published as the *Committee Report and Recommendations: Services to Emotionally Disturbed Children in Saskatchewan.*[92] The committee was made up of senior officials and practitioners from health, education and social services. The members took a broad approach to identifying the problems and made a number of very specific recommendations about how services should be provided in the future.

The committee report noted that since 1950 improvements had been made in services and emphasized the need for prevention and early detection of problems. The committee recognized the importance of the family as the basic social unit and the role of the school as uniquely important to children. The report emphasized the need for increased cooperation and coordination among service providers as was the importance of public education. Highest priority was given to increased medically oriented treatment for youngsters. Interestingly, these same themes still form a major part of every report that is written about the needs of children and youth for health and social services.

The report provided some data on the services that were available and the utilization of services that makes interesting background for this history.

In 1964 Psychiatric Services Branch had outpatient clinics in Saskatoon, Regina, Swift Current, Yorkton, Prince Albert and University Hospital and traveling clinics to 15 locations, as well as the mental hospital facilities in Weyburn and North Battleford.

There were educational psychologists in 7 of the 12 health regions as well as employed by the Saskatoon and Regina School Boards. The Department of Social Services and Rehabilitation operated Embury House, a treatment centre for emotionally disturbed children and Kilburn Hall in Saskatoon and Dales House in Regina provided residential care for troubled youngsters who were hard to place in the foster home system. And there was Saskatchewan Boys' School, a residential program for delinquent boys.

The Report provided the following information:

NUMBER OF DISTURBED CHILDREN SEEN BY PSYCHIATRIC
SERVICES BRANCH IN THE FOUR YEAR PERIOD FROM
DECEMBER 3, 1957 TO 1961.

	Outpatients	Inpatients
University Hospital	332	85
MacNeill Clinic	1490	
Munroe Clinic	1145	18
Moose Jaw Clinic	380	28
Hospital North Battleford	329	15
Hospital Weyburn	146	54
Sask Training School	60	40
Total	**3882**	**240**

Breaking this down, between 1957 and 1961 in the Psychiatric Services Branch outpatient clinics the average number of children and youth seen as outpatients per month at each location was as follows: University Hospital 7, MacNeill Clinic 31, Regina 23, Moose Jaw 8, North Battleford 7 and Weyburn 9. During this four year period, in the entire province an average of 4 youth per month were admitted for inpatient care. Availability of services to youngsters was entirely dependent upon the interests of those who were hired to work in the outpatient clinics. For example, in Regina, in 1967 only one staff member, a speech therapist, was regularly seeing outpatients as the other staff member had resigned and not been replaced.

As well, the report provided data on service utilization in facilities operated by the Department of Social Services. Between April 1960 and March 1962 Embury House provided services to boys who were classed as emotionally disturbed and it received 48 applications for services and 15 of them were admitted.

There were 18 youth discharged during this time. Saskatchewan Boys' School, an institution for delinquent boys, admitted 92 youth with a further 30 in the holding unit. Of these, 18 were deemed in need of treatment and 10 were admitted to psychiatric units. In this same two year period, 23 girls and two boys were placed for residential care out of province in Winnipeg.

The report noted that using the estimates made by the Winnipeg Child Guidance Clinic (10% of all youngsters were classified as having an emotional disturbance) Saskatchewan would have approximately 20,000 youngsters in need of special services. On this basis, the authors recommended an increase of 50 staff in the outpatient clinics. Desirable staffing for each clinic was seen to be 2 psychiatrists, 2 social workers and 1 psychologist. Each clinic was also to have a speech therapist. As well as maintaining Embury House to serve preteen age children and the Saskatchewan Boys' School for delinquent boys, the report concluded that Kilburn Hall and Dales House should remain open and develop specialization in resocialization for younger children as well as providing treatment services for girls. Furthermore, the report recommends that 2 inpatient treatment units be established, each providing 32 treatment spaces and 5 assessment spaces. Desirable staffing for each would be 6 psychiatrists, 6 psychologists, 6 psychiatric social workers, 12 nurses, 75 childcare attendants and 6 teachers.

As well as recommendations to build service capacity, the report emphasized the importance of preventive services in the schools. This is often recommended and seldom acted upon.

The report also called for the establishment of a School of Social Work in the province. One was eventually established in the 1970s. Two recommendations that would certainly be controversial now were to study the possibility of placing Indian and Métis children in white homes for adoption and to broaden the Child Welfare Act to include a new category for intervention called lasting personality damage. In effect, this would have provided a child welfare system for youngsters who were primary mental health clients. The recommendation was not implemented.

The report did not make recommendations about increased public health nursing or educational psychologists. The sweeping changes in special education services that were made in the early 1970s were not foreseen by the report.

In the 1970s Saskatchewan did push forward with the AIM (Adopt Indian and Métis) Program which saw many youngsters placed for adoption in homes outside their culture. This approach had mixed success and was not supported by Aboriginal people or their governments.

The outcome of the committee report was disappointing to all. A part of the problem was timing. The report was released in 1964 in the same year as a government change. Ross Thatcher's Liberals defeated the CCF/NDP. Lawson, who was Director of the Psychiatric Services Branch and had been a member of the committee, resigned soon after the election. The continuity of leadership might have made a difference had he stayed as his work with the committee might have translated into new program developments.

An early decision by the new government was to close

Embury House due to questions about its cost-effectiveness.[93] This decision removed the sole residential component in the overall system of services. The outcome was that many youth were placed out of province for residential care and in the late 1960s the development of Browndale in Moose Jaw and Ranch Ehrlo in Regina.

STATUS OF MENTAL HEALTH SERVICES IN THE 1960s

Mental health services led by the Psychiatric Services Branch remained focused on the problems of the large mental hospitals. Deinstitutionalization took up most of the available manpower, thought and money for the next decade. The continued lack of emphasis on children's services within the Psychiatric Services Branch is a criticism that the architects of the Saskatchewan Plan articulated. Colin Smith as provincial Director of Psychiatric Services wrote,

> "[T]he Saskatchewan program remains essentially an adult one. There is need for greatly improved programs for disturbed children and adolescents." [94]

The lag in development of services to children in Saskatchewan between 1950 and 1970 has been attributed to several primary factors within the Psychiatric Services Branch:

> "The Saskatchewan Plan created an adult community mental health service to replace an adult institutional service. The sheer magnitude of the task of depopulating the institutions and the virtual absence of staff with appropriate training caused the lag in development of children's services." [95]

In Saskatchewan the child guidance clinic model was developed gradually by expansion of the mandates of the outpatient mental health clinics that had developed during the 1960s. This was due in part to continuing lack of trained child psychiatrists. As a general rule admission to hospital was seldom available even for older youth except for those diagnosed with early schizophrenia or demonstrating suicidal behaviour.

It is important to note that the Psychiatric Services Branch was administered by psychiatrists centrally and regionally and did not provide support or leadership to develop a child guidance approach to services nor did they aggressively recruit child psychiatrists. Indeed, services for children and youth were seldom discussed in any planning documents or at meetings.

By 1967, each of the eight regions of the Psychiatric Services Branch had developed outpatient mental health clinics associated with either the general hospital psychiatric ward or with the former mental hospital in Weyburn or North Battleford. Each clinic was staffed by psychiatrists, social workers, community psychiatric nurses and at least one psychologist. The primary responsibility of the clinics was to provide follow-up in the community for patients discharged from the mental hospital or from a general hospital psychiatric ward. Children and youth were seen on referral, usually from schools or general practitioners. However, there was no clear mandate to provide services to youngsters and the provision of services depended largely on the interests and training of individual staff members.

In 1967 a serious incident had a major effect on the provincial program. In August of that year a recently released patient from the North Battleford hospital murdered a family of 9 people in the small community of Shell Lake. This resulted in a report on the Saskatchewan program by Shervert Frazier and his associate Alex Pokorny of Texas. They conducted a series of public and private meetings throughout the province and wrote a report reviewing the Saskatchewan program. Frazier points out that in the first 11 months of 1967 the province lost 17 senior psychiatrists as well as some juniors; the number of social workers was halved from 26 to 13 and several psychologists resigned. He pointed out the causes of these problems in strong terms:

"One of the most recent influences has been a gradual financial squeeze on the Branch. Salaries have fallen behind,
and the leaders of the program have begun to leave. As a
result, quality of care is slipping, caseloads are increasing,
and work days are becoming longer, all contributing to
demoralization. At the present time the personnel situation
is of crisis proportions and must be given first priority."[96]

Frazier recommended significant salary increases for mental health professionals. However concern about the lack of
finances is referred to by Dickinson when he quotes the director of the Psychiatric Services Branch in a memorandum to
the Minister of Public Health regarding hiring a consulting
firm from Winnipeg to recommend follow-up to the Frazier
report so that the "most important recommendations (could)
be implemented by better organization of existing resources."
The response to Frazier was to be to create a better organization rather than provide additional resources.[97]

While Frazier's report was focused in the main on deinstitutionalization and adult programs, he did note that children's
services are inadequate but he made only a weak response:
"We also recommend that appropriate provisions be made
for children, adolescents, alcoholics, addicts, psychopaths and
seniles."[98]

During the 1970s, in the absence of any central policy or
thrust toward the creation of a stronger mental health service for children, regions began to develop programs on their
own initiative with little overall policy direction. This pattern
of resource development has resulted in children's services
being described as "the deprived child"[99] of mental health and
has been the usual pattern in most jurisdictions. Like Topsy,
mental health services for children and youth "just grew."
Certainly in Saskatchewan, the priority given to services for
youngsters varied considerably by region.

The Psychiatric Services Branch central management
structure consisted of a psychiatrist as executive director and
directors of social work, psychology, and nursing along with
parallel professional departments in the regions.[100] Given the

management structure and the historical priorities of the Branch there was no thrust towards a specialized mental health service for children.

SPECIAL EDUCATION IN SASKATCHEWAN

Saskatchewan was the first province to legislate a right to education for all children.[101] This was of major significance and was later copied by other provinces. In 1971 to meet the educational needs of the special student as outlined in the CELDIC report *(see Chapter 2)* the Government of Saskatchewan passed Section 122 of the *School Act* which mandated the provision of special education services. This legislation ensured special class services for youngsters with physical, mental, social and emotional disabilities by requiring local school boards to provide or purchase appropriate services for them.[102] This was a legislated right to education. The majority of youngsters designated as handicapped and thus in need of special services benefited greatly from the legislation.

But the new legislation brought with it a new set of problems as well. The lack of clearly defined criteria for designation, especially of emotional and social handicaps became a major problem.

Some educational administrators required that only psychiatrists could make such designations. At the time, there were only three psychiatrists in the province identified as child psychiatrists – one in Regina and two in Saskatoon. For several years the requirement neatly served to limit the number of youngsters designated.

Children with mental health problems were generally designated as having behavioural problems or were grouped in classes with those whose behaviour was a problem to the school. In many instances, grouping those with mental health problems with those with primary behavioural problems was not a successful form of intervention. The two groups were not compatible in the classroom. In addition, except for young people with physical disabilities there was little attention paid to the needs of high school-aged students. As a result, many teens with emotional or mental health problems left school without completing grade twelve.

The legislation and its regulations mandated that instruction for the handicapped could be provided in resource rooms, special classes or by itinerant teachers. This prescriptive approach to services had many problems. Two examples will assist the reader to understand the problems and to some extent to understand the prevailing lack of understanding of youngsters with emotional or behavioural disorders.

One child was designated as emotionally handicapped on the basis of general misbehaviour and two instances of alleged serious misbehaviour that had not been witnessed by school staff and took place out of school. When a plan was put forward to place the child in another school jurisdiction in a regular classroom with extra assistance to the teacher and individual and family therapy was suggested, the designating superintendent could not agree to the plan as it was deemed to be "not special enough."

Plans were made for another youngster to receive one hour of tutoring a day from the classroom teacher while the class was taught by a qualified substitute teacher. The costs were to be borne by his designation as handicapped. The plan was based on the premise that the special tutoring relationship that would limit the number of adults in the youth's life would generalize into the classroom. But as there was no special classroom and no itinerant teacher involved the plan was deemed unacceptable even though the classroom teacher having taken the required specialized training was qualified under the regulations to provide special services.

A designation as handicapped brought with it special funding for the child in school. However, the primary intervention was to establish special classes and this frequently meant that the child was unable to remain in the local school and had to be transported to the special class or had to leave the school and home to live in another community most often in a city to access special education. There was no infrastructure in place to assist the child living away from home except that available through the Department of Social Services and Rehabilitation which tended not to be involved unless neglect or abuse was an issue. An extra burden of worry for parents who felt pressured to agree to a special class placement in another community was the need to find a suitable boarding house for the child.

CHILD PROTECTION

After the Second World War formal child protection services developed in Saskatchewan. During the 1950s services were delivered through a regional structure and each region assumed responsibility for child protection, adoptions, unwed mothers and juvenile delinquents. Later, the regional offices assumed responsibility for income assistance.

In the early 1960s, as well as providing local community services through the regional offices, the Department of Social Welfare and Rehabilitation operated the Boys' School in Regina a residential school for delinquents and took over responsibility for Kilburn Hall in Saskatoon and Dale's house in Regina. The latter institutions had been operated as children's homes or receiving homes by nongovernmental agencies. There was a mix of youngsters in care in the two institutions – young children awaiting adoption, older youngsters who had been abandoned or had no place to live as they did not fit into foster homes and youth placed in care rather than being treated as juvenile delinquents (often because of a developmental disability). During the 1960s the child protection mandate was strengthened and Dale's house and Kilburn Hall began to specialize more as assessment and treatment units for troubled youth. Prior to this development, youth were often placed in residential treatment centres out of province primarily in Winnipeg and Edmonton. In 1974 the Department of Social Services and Rehabilitation took over responsibility for services for people who were mentally retarded and developed a province-wide regional system of care along with a responsibility for institutional programs.

With the aid of federal cost-sharing the Department of Social Services and Rehabilitation with their child protection mandate developed a strong community program focused on the needs of families and troubled children and youth. Home support services, foster care and residential treatment were developed. On the whole, the department was seen by government to be the locus of responsibility for services to children and youth.

RESIDENTIAL TREATMENT SERVICES

In Saskatchewan, as in other provinces during the 1960s, residential treatment services were established to serve youngsters with emotional and behavioural problems. In the absence of any outpatient community services to provide support, troubled and troubling youngsters were often found to be too difficult for placement in foster homes and a more intensive option was needed.

Following the change in government in 1964, Ross Thatcher's new Liberal government closed Embury House as a cost-effectiveness measure.[103] As this was the only residential treatment program in the province, youngsters were then placed out of province in Winnipeg and Edmonton. At the same time, changed roles at Kilburn Hall and Dale's House provided increased short term assessment and treatment services in Saskatoon and Regina. The child welfare authorities began to work with John Brown, a social worker who had developed residential treatment centres in Ontario. He opened Browndale Residential Treatment Centre in Moose Jaw which operated a series of staffed group homes and served youth with emotional and behavioural disorders. The majority of youngsters were referred for residential care by the Department of Social Services and Rehabilitation through the child welfare mechanism, although, by the early 1970s four youngsters were financed through the Ministry of Health.

A case review of youngsters funded by the Ministry of Health was conducted by James Chapman and Terry Russell of the Regina Region. It proved impossible to achieve a cooperative approach to providing care with the Browndale staff and as a consequence the four youngsters were removed from Browndale and placed in their own homes with support services or in specially trained foster homes in their original communities. As a result of the successful transition back to their own communities of the four children funded by the Department of Health, Al Westcott, Assistant Deputy and Cy McDonald, Minister of Social Services, who were responsible for the remaining youngsters in Browndale asked for assistance to develop a specialized foster home program to be operated in the social service regions. As a result, Browndale was closed in the early 1970s.

In April 1966 Dr. Geoff Pawson established Ranch Ehrlo just outside Regina at Pilot Butte. A private non-profit residential treatment centre for youth with emotional and behavioural problems, Ranch Ehrlo went on to develop a series of staffed group homes in Regina with a board of directors representing the community.

Over the next 40 years Ranch Ehrlo became the largest and most stable residential treatment program in Saskatchewan establishing a Prince Albert campus in 1997 and a Saskatoon campus in 2004, as well as a range of community counselling, housing and recreational services. In 1995 Ehrlo Community Services began providing community based prevention and intervention services. At the time of writing, they were operating four programs in the areas of housing, sports and recreation, counselling and economic development.

A third residential treatment program operated in Regina from the mid-1970s to the 1980s. Bosco Homes sought to differentiate their services from Ranch Ehrlo by focusing on youth with emotional disorders rather than behavioural problems. Ministry of Health funding for youth was stopped following a series of troubling incidents – a death by suicide, a near drowning associated with lax supervision and an allegation of sexual abuse made against one of the staff by a youth. Several years later the program ceased operating in Saskatchewan.

IN SUMMARY

By the end of the 1960s the Saskatchewan public health system was responsible for preventive services through public health nursing, treatment services of speech therapy and audiology, and each regional office had an educational psychologist concerned with early identification and supporting youngsters in schools. The beginnings of specialized mental health services for children and youth were developing as part of the adult mental health system. Child protection, services for delinquents and income assistance were grouped in the Ministry of Social Services and Rehabilitation and it operated or funded foster homes and residential treatment centres. The education system was establishing a strong special education network and in 1970 the new special education legislation was in place and being implemented.

Each system had separate administrations and different regional boundaries. Each system had a separate mandate and was operated by separate professions. Working together on behalf of youngsters in planning and delivering services was totally dependent upon the goodwill of those in the systems. As CELDIC pointed out it did not always work well.

It is of historical interest to note that The Co-coordinating Council on Rehabilitation Annual Congress in 1969 suggested that the council be designated by government as the "new home" of children's services in Saskatchewan. Up to this time the Council had functioned as a central government agency that worked as a vehicle to bring together the various agencies concerned with physical rehabilitation. While the Council provided strong advocacy for member agencies under the leadership of Alan Roehr, various attempts to broaden its mandate, for example, by bringing services for children and at other times services for those with mental retardation into the fold, never came to fruition. Roehr went on to provide national leadership in the field of mental retardation and brought to Canada the concept of normalization that was to revolutionize care for the mentally retarded. One can only wonder what changes would have been made in Saskatchewan's services for children and youth had they been brought together in 1969 under one administration.

5

The Beginnings of a New Program

During the 1960s and 1970s people wrote reports, created committees and held meetings to move the province closer to dedicated mental health services for children and young people. The two decades were marked by inter-professional rivalry and turf battles. There was little clarity about whether the direction should be towards a child guidance clinic model or a child psychiatry model. There was limited leadership from the Psychiatric Services Branch. And, as in the past, there was no active advocacy group in the province pushing for better services for children.

In 1967 an adult mental health clinic was established in Saskatoon and the MacNeill Clinic began to function solely as a children's clinic. In the autumn of 1968 the first child and youth program was established in Regina with a staff of four – social worker, psychologist, speech therapist, reading therapist and a part time consultant psychiatrist. Gradually over the next decade, specialized staff began to be identified in the other eight regions although for many years the team members were assigned only part time to work with youngsters.

A brief paper by Russell[104] written for Dr. James Chapman, then Regional Director of Psychiatric Services in Regina was the first attempt to define the role of the Psychiatric Services Branch in providing services to children and youth. Russell argued that it doesn't make sense to define the service delivery system in the name of professions – psychiatry, social work, psychology, special education.

He proposed that the Psychiatric Services Branch establish core mental health teams for children and youth in each region and that their task be defined as working with other agencies in the community on behalf of youngsters and their families.

These teams were not intended as a separate system, rather one that worked with the other systems to assess problems, define treatment plans and ensure that services were available in the community close to home. In this plan, Saskatoon and Regina were to act as specialist centres providing leadership in the development of services in the other regions and clinical backup as required. The focus of the service would be to provide consultation to other sectors – schools, hospitals, social services, and community agencies. A brief implementation plan for the southern half of the province was included in the paper.

There are two features to Russell's paper that are important to note because they defined for the future the type of mental health service that would develop in Saskatchewan. The paper called first for a multi-disciplinary clinical approach, wherein two or more professionals brought their particular skills to assessment and treatment, and second, for a community building approach, working together on behalf of other systems, providing consultation and assisting them to address problems. These are the predominant characteristics that underscore the development of a child and youth mental health system based in a child guidance clinic model rather than a child psychiatry model based in and growing from a hospital location. In the Psychiatric Services Branch of the 1960s, the predominant model upon which services were based was community psychiatry which, like the child psychiatry model, is dependent for its strength capacity on the availability of hospital beds, psychiatric leadership and services in the community designed specially to support people with mental disorders. The child guidance model seeks to support youngsters at home, in schools and in other systems rather than develop special residential or school facilities for those who are emotionally disturbed or those with mental disorders.

It will not surprise the reader that the development of a child and youth mental health service based in a child guidance or community strengthening approach was not well understood by those responsible for administering Psychiatric Services Branch with its clear focus on psychiatric services for adults and the provision of hospital beds.

ANNUAL CLINICAL CONFERENCE

At this time, the Psychiatric Services Branch regularly held an Annual Clinical Conference attended by many staff members. This event provided opportunities for in-service education and was the main forum for presenting and discussing innovations. Traditionally, it was held just outside Fort Qu'Appelle and was known as The Rally in the Valley. In the late sixties the Branch began to use themes for the deliberations and the meetings began to be hosted in the regional centres.

In 1971 the main theme was mental retardation and the Beddie Report was first on the agenda. Services for mentally retarded people were, at this time, the responsibility of the Psychiatric Services Branch and were delivered mainly through residential care in two institutions, Valley View Centre in Moose Jaw and North Park Centre in Prince Albert. Dr. Alastair Beddie, the Director of Valleyview, argued for changes in services for the mentally retarded to raise the profile of the service and for the establishment of a community program in each region.

A second important presenter at the conference was Dr. Jim Asselstine from the Winnipeg Child Guidance Clinic to discussing his recent report on Children's Services in Saskatchewan. The report was published later that year as "The Three Year Development Plan for Services to Children and Adolescents."[105] The report was written for the Psychiatric Services Branch but no copies have been found. All references to the paper are from other documents. The next mention of this report in the documents available was three years later when Russell summarized the report at the Clinical Conference of 1974 *(see below)*.

Following the 1971 Clinical Conference the staff in mental retardation services and those providing children's services were convinced that the tide was turning and that their services would now receive greater priority. One year later, mental retardation services were transferred from the Ministry of Health to the Core Services administration in the Department of Social Services and Rehabilitation. They were soon to develop a strong network of community based services throughout the province partly due to the federal/provincial cost-sharing agreements negotiated on the social service side. There was no change for services for children and youth.

In late 1972 an Ad Hoc Committee on Psychiatric Team Structure was established with the hope of restructuring professional roles within the Branch. For those who are interested in more details, the ongoing wars among the mental health professions in Saskatchewan during this time have been well documented in *The Two Psychiatries*.[106] The Ad Hoc Report[107] was completed in May 1973 and released by Dr. Louis Skoll, then Deputy Minister in August of the same year. In October 1973 staff of the branch met in North Battleford at the Annual Clinical Conference to continue deliberations towards a new structure for the branch through study of the Ad Hoc Committee Report. Dr. Graham Clarkson, now Deputy Minister, told the gathering that there was no need for new legislation to define the roles of professionals in the psychiatric service, that there would always be a role for the paramedical professions in the Psychiatric Services Branch.

However he made it painfully clear that the paramedical professions would not have a role equal to that of the psychiatrists. This was translated into policy on January 28, 1974 via a long memo from Colin Smith who was now the Executive Director of the Banch.[108] The outcome of several years of angry discussion was a clear statement of the pre-eminence of psychiatry in the system as a whole.

At the Annual Clinical Conference in Yorkton in 1974 the theme was "The Saskatchewan Plan: A Decade in Review and a Look into the Future." While not on the formal agenda, Terry Russell created an opportunity to summarize the results of Asselstine's Three Year Plan for services to children and adolescents in the context of the main concern of the conference – the Saskatchewan Plan which was focused on the needs of the adult psychiatric patient. While the branch had received Asselstine's plan, it was clearly not branch policy and not considered a part of the Saskatchewan Plan. Colin Smith, Executive Director of the Branch in 1973 wrote "...[T]he Saskatchewan program remains essentially an adult one. There is need for greatly improved programs for disturbed children and adolescents."[109] Smith, a psychiatrist, talks about the need for programs for disturbed children and adolescents, not about the need to develop a mental health service for children and families. That is, a child psychiatry model. Russell summarizes the current status of mental health services for youngsters,

"Children's services have grown hardly at all throughout the province. Regions which have been hospital-bed oriented have the lowest number of children registered as out-patients expressed as the percentage of all outpatient registrations for the last six years – (North Battleford 0 to 10.9 and the higher number is for 1968), (Weyburn 4.4 to 6.9) (Moose Jaw 7.1 to 10.5). For the year 1973 these same regions had very low percentages of the estimated populations, 0 – 19 registered (North Battleford .32%) (Weyburn .21%) (Moose Jaw .52%). Using this comparison, Moose Jaw is ahead of Swift Current .42% and Prince Albert .45%. Regina and Saskatoon using the figures of

Harding House and MacNeill Clinic only managed to see 1.18% and .70% of the population." [110]

According to the Asselstine plan there should have been 25 new positions for child and youth services in the province. The reality was 16 positions one of which was a transfer and a second one was a consolidation of two part time positions.

PROBLEMS WITH THE PROVISION OF SERVICES TO CHILDREN AND ADULTS (1974)

In 1974 the Department of Public Health established The Thrust Group. This was a wide ranging planning mechanism whose purpose was to ensure that the NDP policy handbook, used in the 1971 election, was implemented by the Department. At the request of the Thrust Group, an interdepartmental sub-committee of Dave Treherne from Community Health, Terry Russell from Psychiatric Services and David Kelly from the Policy Research Branch prepared a paper outlining the problems with the provision of services to children and adolescents.[111] The report outlined a series of pervasive problems. This report was the first attempt to evaluate the status of community health programs for children and youth and to consider bringing together the services operated by the Psychiatric Services Branch with those of the Community Health Services Branch. The systemic problems outlined by the report included:

- Existing services were not equally distributed across the province. Rural areas were under served. For example, five of ten public health regions did not have a speech therapist, while Yorkton had two, one in each of the Health Region and Psychiatric Services.

- Many planned services were unavailable because of staff shortages. The staff/population ratios of the professions varied widely from region to region. No attempt had been made to estimate and plan for desirable staff/population ratios.

- Services to emotionally disturbed children and adolescents were in particularly short supply.

- Services to children and adolescents were poorly coordinated. Services were administered through a multitude of regional and local units whose boundaries were not co-terminus.

- Services were not uniformly oriented toward work with children and adolescents. Most psychiatric outpatient clinics were providing only limited therapeutic service to children. Only at the newly named Harding House in Regina and MacNeill Clinic in Saskatoon was there access to the full professional complement for a children's mental health team. Elsewhere services were provided by staff that were employed to work in adult psychiatry and had little expertise in working with children. The five child psychiatrists practicing in Saskatchewan were all located in Saskatoon.

- Existing administrative arrangements failed to take full advantage of the Health Region Boards and District Health Councils that could have provided some community participation in planning and direction of services.

- The abilities of front line staff in the community were underutilized, e.g., public health nurses, teachers and social workers.

- The legislation, regulations and administrative procedures of the Departments of Health, Education and Social Services encouraged duplication and fragmentation of services.

- The university training system for professionals which

is "profession-specific" encourages fragmented planning and service delivery.

- Services to youngsters were viewed in isolation from services to the entire family unit.

Further, the Thrust document identifies program inadequacies in four broad areas of service delivery:

- Health Promotion,

- Screening,

- Consultation and Remediation and

- Residential services.

The lack of provincial policy and planning both centrally and regionally was described as the basis of the problems in service delivery.

The Thrust Group had asked the authors to outline the problems in service delivery. The authors outlined some next steps for consideration as well:

- that the Department of Public Health needed to commit to the concepts of comprehensive, multidisciplinary, regionally based and community-oriented services.

- that the Department needed to commit to an operational planning committee to develop the specific policies and procedures necessary to permit the introduction of a child and adolescent service based on the service delivery principles outlined above and

- that within government, a high profile interdepartmental task force should be set up with Ministerial authority to recommend ways in which services could be brought together in a comprehensive manner.

The Thrust Group made minimal response to the paper. Each branch of the Department continued to emphasize the importance of the programs for which they were responsible. There was no advocacy organization in the community pushing for services to youngsters with emotional and behavioural problems. The Thrust Group made recommendations for new program activities involving a dental plan for children, a drug plan, aids to independent living and health promotion. All were implemented by the NDP government of the day.

Due to the lack of response by the Thrust Group, in the same year Russell circulated a proposed planning document within the Psychiatric Services Branch titled, *The Development of Consultative Mental Health Services to Children and Families.*[112] The report followed from the Treherne, Russell and Kelly report. The planning document outlined ways to identify, strengthen and coordinate services provided by the Psychiatric Services Branch. For twenty years, the predominant activity of the eight regions of the Psychiatric Services Branch had been to develop regionalized services for mentally ill adults. However, little had been done to resolve the problem of an effective service system for children and families. Russell's planning document was received but there was no immediate response.

THE 1974 PLANNING REPORT

While there had been national planning documents pertinent to the development of mental health services to children and youth including The CELDIC Report, *One Million Children,*[113] and in Saskatchewan with the *Committee Report and Recommendations: Services to Emotionally Disturbed Children in Saskatchewan,*[114] and *The Three Year Development Plan for Services to Children and Adolescents,*[115] there had been little action to implement new services.

In the Planning Report, Russell identified a number of pervasive problems facing any attempt to develop mental health services for youngsters. The goals of the services provided by the Branch to children and families were diffuse, uncertain and confusing due to inconsistencies between regional administrations, unclear central policy, a lack of clarity of mandate, and the existence of legislation and policy framed to deal with the mentally ill adult.

Divided loyalties were an ongoing problem as individual staff members were asked to apportion their time between child and adult services. This situation was further complicated during the 1960s and 1970s by ongoing conflicts between the professional disciplines that were jockeying for power as described by Dickinson.[116]

The identity and public image of the program was always in question. Public acceptance and perceived relevance and approachability are essential to a strong service. In most instances the image of adult services and the physical base of the facility were described as non-normative and counter productive for the development of services to children and families.

Russell described community mental health services for the young as having little in common with hospital-based services for the mentally ill. Significant areas of difference included: referral sources and contacts, professional colleagues, in-service education needs and the lack of child specific legislation, policy and practice.

Russell provided statistical summary charts based on client contact data for the years 1968 to 1973 for all eight regions. The data showed no consistent growth in services except in Regina and Saskatoon where there were dedicated staff providing the services. Further, where services to children and youth were organized and staffed separately from adult services it was much more likely that a child would be seen in the region of residence.

The recent history of planning for services to children and youth was summarized by Russell. Earlier, in April 1973 prior to the creation of the Thrust Committee, the Branch had set up a series of interlocking committees in an attempt to oversee the development of regional resources, specialized consultation services through resource centres at MacNeill Clinic and Harding House and provincial level planning, program development and evaluation. The results were not promising:

"While this structure has probably increased the commonality of approach between regions and discrete tasks have been accomplished such as the development of policy concerning the purchase of residential treatment, it has not provided for a meaningful thrust in the development of services to children. It is obvious that more structure is needed than intra- and inter- regional coordinating committees with no clear mandate or responsibility and few, if any permanent staff assignments."[117]

The Russell proposal emphasized the underlying philosophy of the changes needed to develop an effective service for youngsters and their families. It was suggested that the branch develop services that were regionally administered, community based, integrated with other services to the maximum extent possible and that utilized institutions as little as possible. He proposed regional consulting teams to work closely with others to multiply the effect of highly trained staff. They were to be "catalysts of problem-solving rather than the sole implementer of palliative measures." If children are to be treated and maintained in their usual or normal environment, those responsible for their care (parents, teachers, social services) must be able to call upon and use adequate consultation and support from staff with highly specialized training.

The planning paper made nine proposals for change in order to operationalize a consulting mental health service for children and families:

- Create a Services to Children and Families Division within Psychiatric Services Branch and appoint an executive director

- Develop strong resource or consulting centres in Regina and Saskatoon

- Create a separate identity in each region and identify staff who work with children and families

- Provide administrative, supervisory and operational direction from the consulting centres in Saskatoon and Regina.

- All staff hired would initially be trained in the consultation centres before becoming operational in the regions.

- Immediate action should be taken to establish local public or consumer participation in planning and operation of regional services by involving local interest groups.

- Adequate staffing was proposed to be a minimum of .5 psychiatrist, 1 psychologist, 1 social worker, 1 psychiatric nurse, 1 speech therapist, 1 reading therapist and 2 clerical staff per 40,000 population.

- All staff of the Services to Children and Families Division would come under a separate sub-vote with regional cost centres so that resources are identified and it is possible to evaluate expenditures against activities.

- It is not necessary to await new budget allocations, rather immediate action should be taken to redeploy existing staff to develop the program.

The 1974 proposal was never implemented. A big stumbling block was the concept of resource centres. Some thought that administering and supervising staff from Saskatoon and Regina wouldn't work – "The distance is too far." Others worried that the city folk wouldn't understand the needs of the rural folk – forgetting that both Saskatoon and Regina had rural populations as well as urban and that many youngsters were being referred to the cities because of the lack of local resources. As well, in regions with only one psychologist they wondered how you could divide him/her up. Nurses and social workers in the regions did not want to lose any of their staff or power to such a move. A further block was the possibility of developing a separate interdisciplinary department. This was perceived as a threat by the existing professional departments. However, the biggest block to implementation was that there was no significant community of interest within the administration of the Psychiatric Services Branch centrally or regionally that was in favour of developing a mental health service for children and youth and no leadership provided by the branch itself.

The absence of central policy direction provided to the developing program in Saskatchewan was an ongoing theme that was further described by Russell and Bell[118] and Bell and Russell[119] in papers delivered to the Western Canada Study Session on Human Services Rural Communities in 1975. "[T]here is some agreement about the foundation, most of us are aware that we are building something. However, little thought has been given to how we are to go about it. Like Topsy, services to children 'just grows.'" Each region in their own way and at different paces had begun to provide services.

The Russell and Bell papers describe in detail the need for a consultative approach that would provide a multiplier effect to the delivery of services

> ". . . . . ..particularly in the rural areas where the interaction of geographic distance and low population density militate against specialized and highly professional services. If children are to be treated and maintained in their normal and usual environment, the people responsible for their care must be able to call upon and use adequate consultation and support from staff with highly specialized training. A consultative team best provides the maximum number of people the benefit of expert knowledge in the least expensive and time consuming fashion."[120]

As they had a large and more varied staff complement, from the beginning the Regina and Saskatoon programs functioned to some extent as resource programs providing consultation to the other regions. It was common for physicians and schools in smaller communities throughout the province to make referrals for diagnostic services.

However, as the rhetoric of the day focused on regional programs, this concept of resource centres was never much recognized. In those days of regional power there was no appetite for centralized resource programs that were likened to the former mental hospitals. The problem in the 1970s was that six of the eight regions did not develop mental health services for children and youth or specialist consulting teams. There was little support for either specialized resource programs or the development of regional services for children and youth.

THE PROVINCIAL CHILD AND YOUTH ADVISORY COMMITTEE

In January of 1978, Dr. Hugh Lafave, the new Executive Director of Psychiatric Services Branch established the Provincial Child and Youth Services Advisory Committee. The purpose "was to devise a mechanism for the development of PSB policy in the area of services to children and families." Membership on the committee was made up of the eight Regional Coordinators of Child and Youth Services. These coordinators were professional staff identified by regional management to attend committee meetings and, in most cases, assume basic responsibility for regional coordination of child and youth services. Only in Regina and Saskatoon were committee members dedicated to children's services on a full time basis; in the other six regions the designate had other clinical and professional responsibilities.

Dr. Garry Bell was seconded from Regina Child and Youth Services to provide leadership.

In an Interim Report prepared by Bell for the committee the following statement reflects the times – "The ultimate goal of this Branch policy is to rationalize the development of services to children and youth without losing sight of regional "differences" and program flexibility.[121] Regional autonomy was clearly in the ascendance and central power as expressed in policy should reinforce "regional differences and program flexibility."

The first task undertaken by the committee was to develop

a set of principles that were to constitute the value base of the program's development.

- Comprehensive – PSB in coordination with other community services should provide the whole range of services beginning with health promotion and screening, and continuing through diagnostic, consultation, remedial, therapeutic and residential services.

- Multi-disciplinary – This service should have within it or have access to all the disciplines which are required to provide services to children, adolescents and families within the PSB. All disciplines which can offer a unique and useful perspective to the overall diagnostic, treatment or service matrix should be involved in an interdependent fashion.

- Regionally-based – The service should be organized and staffed on a regional basis and work towards regional self-sufficiency and accountability.

- Community Oriented – Child and Youth Services should work with and for children and their families in their own community, strive for a high profile and be accessible through open referrals and active outreach.

- Family Centered – Services should support the family as the primary means of assisting the child.

- Early Intervention – Healthy growth and development can best be stimulated early in a child's life. Early detection and intervention should be priorities.

- Continuity of Care – Children and families should experience continuity in the services provided.

- Normalization – Services should facilitate mental health and adhere to the concept of least restrictive alternative.

- Confidentiality – The agency will safeguard the confidentiality of clients and provide access to the family and child (where appropriate) to all information pertinent to the future of the child.

- Informed Consent – It is our obligation to provide information on which the family and/or child might give informed consent for services.

While never formally adopted by the Psychiatric Services Branch, through repetition and usage, these principles became the common philosophical basis for the development of services and are recognized today as underpinning the system of services in Saskatchewan.

The committee summarized their work in this Interim Report as follows: "after five months we have indeed created a viable mechanism for the creation of PSB policy in regards to children and youth. However, in order to derive maximum benefit to the program area it is recommended:

- That a position be created in central office to direct and coordinate the work of the committee and to represent the Branch.

- That mechanisms be explored to recognize and formalize the function of the Regional Coordinator of Youth Services positions such that program area is ensured a strong voice at the regional level.

- That Regional Directors recognize the shortage of staff and take steps to secure more staff or redeploy existing resources.

- That the branch recognize "child and youth" as a priority in the conversion of positions identified via the "Staffing Analysis."

- That the committee assist regions in cooperation with

other agencies to overcome major service gaps – family supports, rural, prevention, early identification, continuum of alternate living resources, consultation, and minority problems."

Representatives from the regions who were involved in providing services to children and youth continued to meet on a fairly regular basis to share information and discuss issues. While there was no mandate for these meetings, there was also no discouragement and so they continued.

SUMMARY OF SERVICE UTILIZATION BY CHILDREN AND YOUTH IN THE 1970s

The size and scope of the problem of mental health services to children and youth were outlined in *Current Health Resources, Organization and Utilation.*[122] The summary of program utilization data for the Psychiatric Branch regional offices that cover the years 1972 to 1978 illustrates the status of service delivery in the eight regional Child and Youth programs:

- Except for University-based facilities the Psychiatric Services Branch provides the majority of available diagnostic, treatment and consultation resources for children with special needs.

- In 1978, the Psychiatric Services Branch provided services to 3,184 children or 1.1% of the population aged 0 to 17.

- At the time, Psychiatric Services Branch services to children and youth were under-developed and poorly distributed by age and location of residence:

- There had been a gradual increase in outpatient services for those aged 0 to 17 and a decrease of inpatient services between 1972 and 1978. The pattern was the same for the Registered Indian Population.

- Services for the young were less available than for adults in all regions.

- The variation in utilization rates per 1000 population varied greatly between regions (6.3 to 16.0).

- All regions except Saskatoon and Regina had rates of less than 10/1000.

- Many youngsters still received services out of their region of residence. The percentage of persons receiving services in their region of residence varied from 61.2% to 99.3%.

- Younger children (0-4) were the least served in all regions even though the rate for 0-4 in the best served region was greater than the rate for all children and youth in the lowest region.

- Older youth are the best served.

- The least well served were those living in unincorporated areas (almost 1/3 of the population)

- The regions that were least well served were the regions that had the largest geographic areas but also the largest budgets because they were the regions that had deinstitutionalized mental hospitals.

The paper outlined several coordination problems resulting from the variation of services available in the regions. For example, there was confusion caused by the lack of consistency in service availability in each region and the lack of central planning and policy to depend upon. The need to develop consultation models rather than depending upon office-based treatment was seen as part of the solution in order to gain a multiplier effect for the services delivered.

So, we end the 1970s. We have the beginnings of child and youth mental health programs in each of the eight regions of the Psychiatric Services Branch. An Interim Committee of Regional Child and Youth Coordinators has identified a value base for provincial program development and made recommendations to branch management regarding organization and staffing but these have not been formally accepted and there is still no provincial program, direction or policy. Topsy still grows at different rates and with different priorities in each region.

6

Regina Child and Youth Services 1968-88

PUTTING THE PRINCIPLES INTO PRACTICE

IN THE BEGINNING

Regina Child and Youth Services (RCYS) was born in November 1968 in the basement of the Regina General Hospital across from the laundry and next to the hospital stores department. Munroe Wing, the inpatient unit was just across the parking lot in a separate building which also housed the adult outpatient department.

The basement space had been previously occupied by the staff of the Outpatient Mental Health Clinic who saw children and their families only if referred. However, there was little emphasis on children's services although there was a speech therapist position which had been vacant for several months. Emmett Hogan, a part time social worker described the dungeon-like atmosphere in a memo to the regional director Dr.

James Chapman . He summarized his comments with the following:

> "The physical structure of this clinic is inadequate in every respect, and is conducive of feelings of apathy on the part of staff who work there, and disbelief on the part of parents who bring their children there for help."[123]

Hogan described the staffing and service provision as chaotic, haphazard and stop-gap with staff borrowed from the adult clinic. He proposed a permanent, staffed facility for children "as the only way to put an end to the manipulating, needling, and criticizing of present children's clinic staff by local doctors."

In Regina, at this time, psychiatric services were delivered through the Munroe Wing and Clinic. The 30 bed in-patient unit was the locus of service and was housed in an old two story building behind Regina General Hospital. In 1931 it became The Psychopathic Ward, Saskatchewan's first non-institutional mental health facility. It was later renamed Munroe Wing after a former Minister of Health and in 1947 the provinces first out-patient services were introduced.

The organizational structure was typical of all Psychiatric Services Branch facilities at the time: a psychiatrist was the director and professional departments – nursing, social work, psychology – reported to him through department heads. This structure, a carry-over from the medical model in use in the two major psychiatric institutions, emphasized the maintenance of medical dominance in terms of professional roles and power. However with the transition to community psychiatry in the 1960s "inter-occupational conflict"[124] became an increasing problem, resulting in fragmentation of service and inter-professional power struggles.

At the provincial level de-institutionalization continued to be the top priority. In four years the mental hospital in Weyburn cut its in-patient population by almost two-thirds – dropping from a head count of 1478 in 1962 to 501 in 1966. Community psychiatry teams had been established in all Psychiatric Services Branch facilities in southern Saskatchewan to support those discharged and to provide services to prevent admissions. As described earlier, exciting research was taking place, services were changing rapidly and the environment seemed open to change.

Dr. James Chapman, the medical director of the Regina Region, had done pioneering work in the diagnosis and care of young schizophrenics in Scotland and was one of the driving forces behind the development of a specialized mental health service for children and youth. The other significant person was Terry Russell, who had just returned from doctoral studies to become the chief psychologist for the region. He had many years of experience working with children at Camp Easter Seal and the Physical Restoration Centre and a lifelong commitment to children and youth. Together the two men provided the impetus and leadership for the development of a specialized program aimed at resolving the concerns identified by Emmett Hogan and others.

From the beginning the staff was multi-disciplinary by design, and comprised a social worker, reading therapist, speech therapist, psychologist, part-time consultant psychiatrist and two clerical staff. As the program developed, the multi-disciplinary nature of the staff continued to develop as well.

The intent was to avoid the inter-professional conflict which permeated the adult mental health facilities and bring a range of perspectives to the amelioration of child and family problems.

Gradually the term interdisciplinary replaced multidisciplinary because it was a better descriptor of the program that evolved. Clinical assessment and treatment for each referral was usually provided by a two person team – one with a child focus and one with a parent or family focus. At referral one team member was designated primary consultant responsible for overall case management and general administration of the file. As the program grew and became differentiated with specializations in early and middle childhood and youth services the interdisciplinary nature of the intake system was continued.

The new child and youth program was almost immediately faced with a high demand for its services. By 1970 the number of referrals had doubled although the staffing complement had not increased beyond the original five. The Branch priority remained the development of adult services to support deinstitutionalization and there was no financial support from the central office in recruiting more staff for children's services. There was little opportunity for growth and creative approaches to staffing – begging, borrowing and even stealing – were required.

The first success was based on a memo from the director, Terry Russell to Joe Dvernichuk, Administrator of the Psychiatric Services Branch pointing out that from 1969 to 1972 35% of the clients registered who lived outside the city of Regina were from the Weyburn Region.[125] The solution was to transfer to Regina one of the Weyburn social work positions and a psychiatrist's salary with the agreement that the Regina program would provide consultation services in southern Saskatchewan. This worked well as youngsters from other southern regions were already being referred, many from the paediatric ward in the Regina General Hospital, and there was considerable demand for Regina staff to participate in clinical hospital consultations.

A second successful creative staffing move followed a joint review with the child welfare authorities of the Browndale Residential Treatment Centre program. The outcome of the review was that Browndale was closed and the residential treatment costs were diverted to establish a position for a psychiatric nurse who then developed community programs for the youngsters who had been at Browndale.

A third successful creative staffing foray resulted from the advocacy of parents of children with autism and related disorders. It was impossible to deliver intensive home-based programs with such a small staff. As well, at this time, there was a freeze on establishing new staff positions in the public service. The result was the development of a new community agency, the Society for the Promotion of Educational Achievement for Children in the Home, (SPEACH) which was operated by a parent--managed board of directors and employed four staff on the basis of a contract with Regina Child and Youth Services.

By 1971 the child and youth staff had increased and the program had outgrown the cramped quarters in the basement of the hospital resulting in professional staff having to share office space.

COMMUNITY ACCESS

Concern about the program's inappropriate location in the basement of the hospital was growing. Staff increases added to the problem and by 1971 there was support for a move.

The Public Works Department had initially encouraged a move to a new eight-story office block on Victoria Avenue just east of Victoria Park. The entire top floor and some space on the floor below were available. It was evident to program staff that being located in an office tower with the head office of the Department of Education and other corporate entities would inhibit access to services and Public Works was urged to look for alternatives. When it was pointed out that play space out -of- doors was required, it seemed that they might have to reconsider their plan. Amazingly, they offered a roof-top playground with all new equipment! This required only a one word response – "suicide" – and the move to Victoria Avenue was squelched.

A much better solution was a move a few blocks away from the hospital to Harding House at 1731 College Avenue at the corner of Broad Street. This large building had formerly been used as a residence by the Qu'Appelle Diocesan School or as it was commonly known, QDS. The chapel was converted to a playroom complete with sandbox and the Director's office had a working fireplace. After this move the program was commonly referred to as Harding House. High marks were accorded the agency for the non-stigmatizing nature of this name in a 1974 program evaluation.[126]

1976 saw another move to a much larger space just two blocks away and Harding House became Child and Youth

Services when the clinic took over the main school building on the former Qu'Appelle Diocesan School property at 1601 College Avenue. Here it remained for the next twenty-eight years, a period of remarkable growth and change for the program. The building provided sufficient private offices, age-appropriate playrooms, a community meeting room, a much improved reception area, ample playground space and free parking for clients and staff. Its unique history, character and location in a park-like setting close to the city centre made it in many ways an ideal space for a program aiming to develop a range of innovative community-oriented services. There was always some unused corner available for students or for a community program in need of meeting space or a short term office, and the castle-like façade, gargoyles and hidden staircases were attractive to children and families. In time, the building known in Regina as QDS for its first 60 years became known as Child and Youth Services.

THE EARLY PHILOSOPHICAL BASIS OF REGINA CHILD AND YOUTH SERVICES

Very early in the development of the new service, a scope paper[127] was developed which became the basis on which services were developed over time. The program was strongly committed to a health emphasis and the basic conviction was that not only can dysfunction be remediated but that it can be prevented. To this end efforts were geared to identify strengths and weaknesses not only within the child but within his family and community as well. Two objectives were established and articulated in an article by David Randall

1. The provision of comprehensive services to ensure the maintenance of and encourage the development of the health, social and educational welfare of children and youth.

2. The provision of all necessary remedial services for all children with special needs – the mentally ill, the

delinquent, the mentally retarded, and other handicapped children and youth.

The objectives were to be pursued by operating with six basic principles upon which the service was founded:

1. Comprehensive – In coordination with other community services, provides the whole range of services beginning with health promotion and screening, and continuing through diagnostic, consultation, remedial, therapeutic and residential services.

2. Multidisciplinary – The service should contain within it or have access to all the disciplines which are required to provide services to children, adolescents and families within the Psychiatric Services Branch. All disciplines which can offer a unique and useful perspective to the overall diagnostic, treatment or service matrix should be involved in an interdependent fashion.

3. Regionally-based – The service should be organized and staffed on a regional basis. It should work toward regional autonomy and accountability. The services should be delivered close to the person's home and family.

4. Community-oriented – The Child and Youth Service should work with and for children and their families in their own communities, by uniting homes, schools and community institutions and services. It should strive for a high profile in the community and be accessible to the public through open referral and active outreach.

5. Family Centred – The services should reflect the conviction that support to the family is a primary means of assisting the child. The intention is to maximize the degree to which any family acts and feels capable of managing its own affairs.

6. Early Intervention – Healthy growth and development can best be stimulated early in a child's life. Therefore early detection and intervention should be a priority throughout Child and Youth Services.

Lofty ideals indeed for a small program with seven staff at the time; however, these have remained the goals that underpin the provision of services to this day.

MAKING INTER-PROFESSIONAL WORK

During the 1970s in Branch facilities throughout the province there was a continual jockeying for power and status among the mental health professions. Teams consisting of a psychiatrist, a social worker and a community nurse were established in developing the program of community psychiatry in the eight regions of the province. Psychiatrists managed the system at the provincial, regional and team levels. In most regions all referrals went first to a psychiatrist who made the decisions about which disciplines would be involved in providing services. However, in some regions direct referrals were made to the various disciplines and this had been the case for several years. In 1972 the Director of the Psychiatric Services Branch, Colin Smith, decided to end this practice and unwittingly escalated the struggle for power. His memo to the Minister of Public Health Walter Smishek outlines the proposed solution. He planned to travel to Weyburn the next day "to rescind this policy [direct referrals to other disciplines] immediately and to make all referrals come to a psychiatrist in the first instance who may assign them as he feels appropriate."[128] This caused a rebellion that resulted in the creation of the Ad Hoc Committee on Psychiatric Team Structure of 1973. These problems have been described in detail by Dickinson in *The Two Psychiatries*.[129]

At RCYS professional supervision was provided by senior clinicians in each profession. However, the organizational emphasis was not on professional departments but rather on program assignment to the early childhood, middle childhood or youth program. Part of the solution to the problem of inter-professional rivalries was shared clinical work and equality of assignment of responsibility as primary case consultant. In order to overcome professional power struggles the power base of the team was dispersed and was called an interdependent team (as opposed to autocratic or autonomous practice team systems).

Clinical teams were created for each case rather than having a team responsible for a number of cases. The clinicians involved made the decisions about the model of service delivery appropriate for each individual case. The question of role conflict was addressed by organizing several disciplines into two large categories, child advocates and family advocates, based on training, interest and expertise. Each individual could specialize on other than professional grounds. Each clinical team had both a child advocate and a family advocate either of whom might be assigned overall responsibility for case management.

Regina Child and Youth Services further de-emphasized professional divisions by emphasizing functional concerns or problem areas.

The second major feature that minimized professional conflict was shared planning for program development, coordination and consultation. As staffing increased and program differentiation evolved, the words used to describe the programs mirrored the interdisciplinary nature of the developing model. Resource collectives were developed and assigned responsibility for coordination with other service providers and for the development of consultation agreements with other agencies in the community. The resource collectives focused on consultation and program development in three main areas: for parents and families, for schools and for youngsters with developmental disabilities. Each staff person was a member of two of these resource collectives, one age based and one program based and was expected to develop formal consultation arrangements with other agencies in the community – day cares, foster homes, special school classrooms, parent groups, and so on. Job descriptions were rewritten to include community development/consultation responsibilities as well as the traditional assessment and treatment roles.

As can be seen from the above description the program, while based in clinical assessment and treatment, was committed to coordination of services with other providers, formal consultation agreements with other agencies, community program development and mental health education. The complexity of relationships with the community was managed by the resource collectives and developed and monitored by individual staff depending upon interest, capacity and time.

Professional staff members whose training was largely clinical in orientation were often uncomfortable with the expectation for community work when first joining the agency. I remember doing a six month evaluation for a new psychologist. She appeared to be most worried about the outcome. When she had passed the evaluation with flying colours, she relaxed and said she thought that she would fail as she only had developed one consultation agreement and she thought I would have expected much more. Between us we agreed that a recent graduate who was a single parent with children at home was doing very well and needn't worry about her performance as a community consultant.

There were many different professional disciplines working together and providing a well-knit interdisciplinary approach to mental health services for children and youth. However, the provincial human resource system had a classification system based on professional departments and could not reward the work that was being done at RCYS with higher classifications and higher salaries. It took many years of lobbying and scores of memos to the personnel branch for them to change their classification system. But gradually the system began to create senior consulting positions in nursing, psychology and social work based on their program specialization and leadership rather than supervision within their discipline. Rather than being the chief social worker or psychologist, it became possible to move to a higher classification when one had responsibility for a targeted program. This was a major breakthrough in personnel classification procedure and made management of and working in an interdisciplinary program an easier and more rewarding task.

COMMUNITY DEVELOPMENT AND CONSULTATION

From its inception, RCYS was a community leader with involvement in many community activities and organizations. There was always an emphasis on consulting with the community and working toward the development of new services to fill gaps in the overall service system. In 1978 after ten years of operation, Bell and Lafave summarized the community consultation and resource development relationships currently in place. "We currently do clinical consulting to seven main line agencies such as school boards, hospitals and Social Service departments. More significantly we provide both program and clinical input to two old and nineteen new service organizations.

Our agency has played a key role in creating the new services and has been the primary thrust behind thirteen of those nineteen."[130]

In discussing community development and outreach services, Bell and Lafave tell us:

> "The uniqueness of our service lies on the one hand in the perspective derived from the value based principles which constitute the ideology of our service. On the other hand we have placed in one system the single most well qualified, diverse and comprehensive cluster of child and family oriented clinical skills in the community. Our open referral policy and diverse range of talents meant that we draw problems from virtually every quarter of our population. Our service thus becomes a hub for both identifying service gaps and coordinating outreach and community resource development activies."[131]

Some examples of the early community development activities of the agency help to tell the story.

REGINA ASSOCIATION FOR CHILDREN
WITH LEARNING DISABILITIES

One of the first examples grew directly out of our clinical work. In the late 1960s learning disability was a relatively new term. Partly as a time saving mechanism because many of the issues were the same for each family, Russell and Bonnie Main decided to establish a therapy group for the parents of children with learning disabilities because while doing clinical work we found ourselves repeating the same information to each family. After two meetings it became clear that the parents did not need therapy. They needed good diagnoses for their youngsters and to learn about self and group advocacy. The result was the establishment of the Regina Association for Children with Learning Disabilities, an organization that played a central role in educating RCYS staff, both local school boards and the Ministry of Education about the changes that were needed to ensure that their children were educated appropriately in schools. Several years later with changes to the school systems RCYS no longer needed a reading therapist and in 1976 the position was converted to that of an educational psychologist and the focus broadened to provide a more complete diagnostic and consultation capacity.

MOBILE FAMILY SERVICES SOCIETY (MFSS)

The initial impetus for bringing together the community agencies that formed MFSS was to obtain federal and provincial funding to launch innovative programs appropriate to the changing lifestyles of youth during the early 1970s. The project funding included employing young people to provide a 24 hour crisis telephone line with appropriate follow up services. The success of this program led to a request from the Department of Social Services to develop a new component geared to providing after hours and weekend crisis responses to children and families where child protection might be an issue.

MFSS provided a 24 hour crisis response service for youngsters and their families. The corporate board of directors was composed of delegate members of twenty-eight community service agencies – mental health, police, child protection, downtown churches, community and social agencies. At the time that the employees unionized, Garry Bell was the first Chairman of the Board of MFSS and was a member of the SGEU, the union that was organizing the staff. It was an amazing balancing act.

REGINA ASSOCIATION FOR AUTISTIC CHILDREN

In the 1960s, youngsters with autism spectrum disorders were generally placed in The Harrow deGroot School (a school for the mentally retarded, as students with developmental disabilities were then known). The school had begun with a parent controlled community board. RCYS made an arrangement to provide diagnostic and consulting services to the school. As part of the children's assessments, the parents were interviewed and many were floundering, overcome with the care of their children. Based on the experience with the Regina Association for Children with Learning Disabilities, we organized a parent information evening that in a few short months developed into the Regina Association for Autistic Children. With the competent leadership of one of the parents, Marion Beck, we assisted the parents to operate home-based summer programs including a camp utilizing summer student grants to train and supervise university students. The Regina Catholic School Board agreed to establish two special classrooms in an elementary school with ample provision for classroom integration and staff provided regular clinical consultation to the school.

In 1977 the group of about thirty parents hosted in Regina the first national conference on children with autism -- a highly successful event. The conference proceedings included expression of family concerns and professional papers. Proceedings were later published.[132]

In the same year the parents incorporated the Society for the Promotion of Educational Achievement for Children in the Home (SPEACH) and thus had a program of regular home and community child care services and respite available to them. SPEACH continues to provide services through a contract with RCYS.

THE DEVELOPMENTAL CENTRE SOCIETY

This was both a centre based day program and a home based program for multiply disabled youngsters. With a community board and parent leadership the organization provided a comprehensive program for youngsters who were not at that time able to attend school as there were no facilities available for them. It was piloted at RCYS and developed into a significant force in the community under the leadership of Clare Parker and June Mitchell. As years went by the program was funded by the Regina School Board and operated as part of the public school system until the target group was incorporated into special education programs.

THE REGINA PARENT EDUCATION ASSOCIATION

In 1972 staff from Child and Youth Services met with Catholic Family Services, the Family Service Bureau and the Department of Social Services to discuss issues around the growing number of referrals of child/family conflict that all agencies were experiencing. Parent education in a group format was emerging in the literature as a useful approach for many families and it was thought that it would be worthwhile to develop this as an option for Regina. As no agency had primary responsibility for prevention it was agreed to band together to form a non-profit organization to develop classes in Regina and involve community groups including churches and community associations. The goal was to pursue a self-help approach in which experienced parents became the group leaders.

The Adlerian approach as interpreted by Dr. Rudolph Dreikers was developed by other authors into a program called Systematic Training for Effective Parenting (STEP)which eventually became widely available at the community level with delivery coordinated through the Regina

Plains Community College. It is estimated that over 2000 parents took the STEP program between 1972 and 1988. Key to its success were the energy and commitment of two women, Louise Sutherland and Rose Stepan, who took one of the first classes offered through Catholic Family Services. They subsequently volunteered thousands of hours to prepare and present classes, find and train other parent leaders, and serve in various executive capacities on the RPEA Board. They also provided leadership to the development of a highly effective group leadership training program which was eventually a regular offering of the community college to train people for a variety of leadership roles.

THE QUIET HIGH SCHOOL DROPOUT

The program was established in 1972 in a classroom in the basement of RCYS to provide school and day programs for youth with early schizophrenia and other serious mental disorders. The name was derived from a brief paper prepared for the school boards to describe the plight of youth with mental illness who seldom were able to stay in school. The school boards agreed to a pilot project and Regina Catholic Schools hired and seconded Tom Riffel as teacher/counsellor to work with the students utilizing correspondence courses and early reintegration in one of the high schools nearby. Bonnie Young and Greg Petroski worked closely with the students helping them to develop life skills in parallel with the new educational opportunities. The program resulted in many fewer readmissions to hospital and provided realistic plans for school re-entry. After several years, the location of the program was moved to a classroom in Miller Collegiate thus making reintegration easier and communication with teachers much more effective.

THE BALFOUR SPECIAL TUTORIAL PROGRAM

Established in 1972, this was the first in any Saskatchewan high school to provide specialized education for pregnant teens. Its existence was due to the commitment of a retired teacher, Alice Perry and a school superintendent with the Regina Board, Alex MacKenzie, who were concerned about the increasing number of young women who dropped out of school due to pregnancy and the high percentage who never returned. Together they convinced the Board to provide a self-contained space with a private entrance at Balfour High School. Shirley Schneider was the first teacher. It was easily accessible and school hours were arranged to maximize privacy of travel on the public system. Students took correspondence classes under teacher supervision. Child and Youth Services, through Laura Carment and later Bonnie Young, provided group discussion and support for students and program development consultation to staff. Public health nurses and social services workers used the site to deliver mandated services. The Special Tutorial became highly successful and served as a model for others in the province and country. Mrs. Schneider was instrumental in developing another first – an off-site infant day care centre operated by a volunteer community board. The day care was named after Alex MacKenzie.

INSTITUTIONAL AND RESIDENTIAL CARE

RCYS prided itself in an approach to services that might be described: Do it now! Do it at home and in the community! Close relationships with the hospital emergency ward and Munroe Wing allowed easy consultation, admission as necessary, and involvement in treatment and discharge planning. Older youth were occasionally placed in approved homes and the operators given training and consultation. When several patients with mental health disorders as well as developmental delays were discharged from Browndale Treatment Centre and Valley View Centre funds were found to hire Bob Scott, a psychiatric nurse, to provide community services. No attempts were made to provide alternative care homes. Rather than develop a parallel care system the staff worked closely with the staff of the Department of Social Services providing direct and consulting assistance to children in care and to foster homes.

As well, there were ongoing efforts to provide services to families to prevent breakdown and subsequent wardship.

EARLY CHILDHOOD SERVICES

From the beginning there was recognition of the need for early childhood services. The development of Resource Collectives that were age-based ensured that there was staff dedicated to serving very young children. It is interesting to note that in many jurisdictions in the new century there is still little emphasis on meeting the mental health needs of the young child. Referral patterns in most jurisdictions show that it isn't until age five and school entry that youngsters are referred. As with the other collectives there was a clinical component and a consulting effort but the main program change initiated by the Early Childhood Collective was to focus the attention of the agency on the need to provide home-based rather than centre-based services.

THE RAINBOW YOUTH CENTRE

The idea of a drop-in centre for youth began as a class project led by a group of social work students at the University of Regina. They established a planning committee involving staff from a variety of community agencies including Child and Youth Services, which agreed to use funds from a vacant staff position on a short-term basis to employ Debbie Pearce as a director/counsellor. The City of Regina offered space in a former dairy building in downtown Regina. A volunteer community board was established and obtained funding initially through creative use of federal grants intended for youth job training. In order to renovate the dairy into a youth centre the grants were used to hire a Vocational Counsellor who was an experienced general contractor and to pay wage subsidies to unemployed youth who were learning about construction work. Later, contracts for renovations were signed with community organizations and individuals and eventually the profits funded a second work crew that cut, hauled and sold firewood. The Drop-In Centre provided after-school and evening programs and the youth involved in employment programs were also expected to take part in evening programs. Over time, youth who had been involved in the program were hired as youth workers (often with the creative use of employment opportunity grants).

By involving youth in all aspects of the program and encouraging their ownership and control of the program Rainbow became a community for youth rather than a place where troubled youth were sent. Over the years programs and services changed according to youth needs, agency location and available funding. The program moved to Dewdney Avenue in the late 1980s and developed a well-attended evening meal program which was widely recognized as an important contribution to the growing concerns about inner-city hunger in Regina. At the same time this location created recognition of the need to incorporate younger clients into service delivery. In the absence of core funding Rainbow continued to depend on grants from organizations such as Health Canada and contracts with local health, social service and education agencies until the mid-1990s when two full time positions were funded through the Mental Health Services Branch. Rainbow subsequently improved its accessibility and programming through a move to a larger youth-oriented building in North Central Regina and in 2007 celebrated 25 years of service to children and youth. In 2007 their budget, with all of their grants, was over one million dollars.

YOUNG OFFENDERS SERVICES

A significant program development occurred in 1984 following the passage of the new Young Offenders Act by the federal government. For the first time, federal cost-sharing of mental health services was made available to ensure that the court-ordered assessments identified in the Act were available. Across Canada differing approaches to service delivery were taken and in Saskatchewan the provincial departments of Social Services, Justice and Health collaborated on the development of these new services and agreed to establish them within the Mental Health Services Branch at their Regina, Saskatoon and North Battleford Child and Youth Facilities. As a result, Regina Child and Youth Services got two specialized psychologists and additional funding for contracted child psychiatry staff to provide assessments ordered by the courts and consultation services to staff of the youth probation and youth custody facilities.

A PROVINCIAL PROGRAM IS BORN

From 1968 to 1982 the programs in Regina and Saskatoon had grown and consolidated but this was not the case in the other regions. Fourteen years is a long time to advocate with little success on behalf of the development of a provincial program.

In the early1980s following several years of discussions the Department of Health agreed to establish a province-wide program of Child and Youth Mental Health Services. Activities leading up to this important decision are described in detail in the following chapter, (chapter 7). New funds were made available in 1982-84 and each of the eight regions developed a core team of workers. Laura Carment left her job as assistant director and chief social worker at RCYS to be the first provincial director. Under her leadership provincial policy was developed and planning proceeded with the assistance of the regional coordinators of child and youth services who now met on a monthly basis.

TROUBLE ON THE HORIZON

The Conservative government of the day was increasingly concerned with the growth of the public service. During their second term of office beginning in 1986 the government initiated two programs to address this problem. Firstly, they introduced a process to limit new hiring and ordered that vacant positions be deleted in order to save salary costs. Second, they instituted a program that encouraged senior staff to opt for special benefits if they would retire earlier than the usual age.

As a result in 1987 Regina Child and Youth Services lost three senior position. RCYS had an almost complete turnover of staff in 1986 and 1987 – 12 of 16 clinical positions. The result for the province as a whole was that most of the gains from 1982 to 1986 were lost.

Additionally, the first director, Terry Russell had resigned in 1986 to move to British Columbia where he became the first provincial director of child and youth mental health services. Russell was replaced as director by a psychiatrist, Dr. Jim Turanski.

In combination, the deletion of three positions and the turnover of 75% of the staff caused massive disruption to the service. Historical continuity was lacking and senior clinical and supervisory skills were sorely missed. As well as attempting to keep up with the clinical referrals, remaining senior staff members were doing double duty supervising new staff many of whom were inexperienced. At this time, requests for service increased considerably in part due to parallel staff cuts in other agencies which were referring clients that they were unable to serve. The general outcome was that agencies in the community became more protective and restrictive – narrowing their referral door in order to try and manage their work. The increased number of referrals was managed in part by providing immediate assessments and having a wait list for therapy. In many instances the practice of interdisciplinary assessment was replaced by assessments carried out by a single staff person.

The program staff working on the Youth Services Team developed an innovative response to the increase in service demand, The Group Intake Program. In this program all families referred were offered the option of attending evening sessions once weekly for three weeks. Each evening opened with family groups working at individual tables under the leadership of a team of therapists to identify their specific concerns through discussion and paper and pencil responses to a questionnaire. This was followed by an educational session on a topic related to family dynamics and communication.

The program aimed to reduce the need for individual therapy. It was successful in reducing wait times for first service from three months to one week and in 1988 received the "Triple E" an award from the Mental Health Services Branch for this achievement. It was discontinued after one year when a program review concluded that the reduction in requests for ongoing therapy were not sufficient to warrant the staffing costs associated with providing evening services.

However, after 1988 when Laura Carment left the provincial director position and returned as director of RCYS the program stabilized and has remained strong ever since. Carment retired in 1997 and was replaced as director by Dr. David Randall. In 2002. Randall retired and was replaced by Joanne Phillips who continues to provide creative leadership until her retirement in 2012.

7

International Year of the Child and International Year of Youth

ORGANIZATIONAL GROWING PAINS

INTERNATIONAL YEAR OF THE CHILD

The United Nations declared 1979 the International Year of the Child. A description of the national perspective is included in chapter 2.

Within the Saskatchewan Government one of the primary activities took place within the Health Department. A year long study was undertaken to examine the health of children and youth in the province, to review the services available to them and to make recommendations for the future. The review team members were Terry Russell of the Psychiatric Services Branch, Jane Aitkena public health nursing consultant, Garry Curtis and Jayne Mihalyko both of the Policy Research and Management Services Branch.

The research project produced four documents which summarized its findings.

- Current Health Resources, Organization and Utilization1[133] was a technical report that described in detail the services for children and youth provided by the Department of Health and the available resources and their utilization. All agencies funded by the Department were included in this study which outlined the legislative or regulatory authority, the objectives and policy, personnel and facilities and the utilization of services. Utilization data were summarized for the years 1972 through 1978.

- Youth, Health and Lifestyles[134] reported on a survey of 738 never-married youth aged 15 – 19. The sample was randomly chosen to represent the age, sex and rural/urban distribution of young people in the province. The survey measured knowledge, attitudes and behaviour in a variety of healthy lifestyle areas including nutrition, smoking, alcohol and drugs, sexuality, family and peer relationships and self-concept. The results provided a baseline of information to develop future health promotion opportunities for young people.

- Learning Though Living Health[135] summarized research and strategies in health promotion and provided a framework for the young to learn about health. The main purpose of the research was to explore how children learn about heath and what motivates the development of healthy lifestyles and decisions. The focus was on informal learning. The findings are reported using an ages and stages format.

- Saskatchewan Health for Children and Youth[136] was the major component of the review and it integrated the results of the other reports, examined the range of health needs and services, and recommended short

term changes, new service thrusts and major organizational changes.

RECOMMENDATIONS OF THE REVIEW OF CHILD AND YOUTH HEALTH SERVICES

On February 16, 1981, the four reports that constituted the
review were released publicly by the Minister, Herman
Rolfes. In releasing the report, Rolfes stated:

> "The Report suggests that we can generally meet the
> physical needs of young people in periods of illness.
> However, we cannot assure them of the opportunity to
> learn and practice good health habits. As well, we cannot
> always ensure that developmental problems will be iden-
> tified and that adequate remedial action will be available
> when and where it is needed. I am convinced that future
> improvements in health status will develop from a better
> balanced and more effectively coordinated service deliv-
> ery structure."[137]

Some results came quickly. Immediate changes included
establishing a school health demonstration project in Moose
Jaw and a province-wide campaign to reduce childhood
injuries. For the purposes of this history, the four volumes of
the review have three important uses. The first is the detailed
analysis of the Psychiatric Services Branch data reporting on
service delivery utilization between 1962 and 1968. The second
is the specific guidance for the delivery of mental health services in Saskatchewan. The third is a series of organizational
recommendations to improve the coordination and delivery
of all health services for children and youth provided by the
Department of Health.

A snapshot of the utilization data shows that from 1972
to 1978 there was an increase in the utilization of outpatient
services in the Psychiatric Services Branch by children and
youth from 2,491 outpatients or 7.7 per 1000 population to

3,184 or 11.0 per 1000 population. In the same years there was a decline in inpatient services from 159 (.05 per 1000) to 100 (.03 per 1000). Youngsters who were registered Indians had lower rates of utilization of outpatient services except for 15 to 19 year olds and higher rates of utilization of inpatient services. However, from 1972 to 1978 youngsters 0 – 17 who were registered Indians increased their utilization of services from 4.6 to 8.4 per 1000 population.

The review recommended that steps be taken to ensure more adequate outpatient services for youngsters who are registered Indians. The analysis also showed generally higher rates of utilization of services by youngsters living in villages.

Consequently, the review recommended that services be provided as close to the place of residence as possible not just in regional centres and that steps be taken to ensure adequate coordination and follow-up when services were provided away from the youngster's home community.

However, by far the most significant recommendations of the review were focused on the organizational and management structure of the Department of Health. In order to ensure effective health services for children and youth in the future, the review outlined three priorities for departmental action

- improving the internal coordination of programs for children and youth

- taking responsibility for establishing preventive services where there is a likelihood of future health costs

- identifying significant areas of contact with other departments and agencies providing services to children and youth and

- committing to coordinated action to solve problems in these areas.

Two main themes were at the core of the review recommendations – themes that were important to everyone who spoke to the review team – problems in coordinating services and the importance of prevention and early intervention to ensure the future health of children and youth.

The organizational recommendations were focused on improvements in service coordination and on ensuring the priority of prevention and early intervention. The three recommendations were that

- Saskatchewan Health should consolidate under Community Health Services Branch the child and youth health services now available at the regional level through CHSB, PSB and the Saskatchewan Alcoholism Commission to form the basic services to be deployed at the regional level.

- The Minister of Health should appoint a high level provincial advisory committee on child and youth health with broad public and professional membership including youth representatives.

- Saskatchewan Health should enact legislation clearly defining the mandate of Saskatchewan Health for the provision of health services to children and youth.

The key to making the changes that were seen to be required was to bring the community health services for children and youth together under one administration whose major focus is prevention and which works in the schools on a regular basis. The provincial advisory committee would be a visible force that would advocate for youngsters who have little voice or power in government decision making. Enacting legislation was seen as a way to build into the fabric of the department the certainty that children's mental health mattered.

It will be no surprise to the reader that a recommendation for such sweeping organizational change caused a great deal of discussion among the branches of the department that would be affected by the proposed changes. The next section describes the aftermath of the report and the responses to the recommendations.

CHILD AND YOUTH SERVICES TASK FORCE – 1981

On January 9, 1981, prior to the release of the report, Ken Fyke, Deputy Minister of Health, established a Child and Youth Services Task Force.[138] Its purpose was to respond to issues identified in the report and to plan the implementation of those decisions by the Department subsequent to the release, discussion and analysis of the recommendations. Fyke established the Task Force as a senior policy body to advise on necessary steps to be taken to improve child health services. The Task Force was co-chaired by Hugh Walker and John Yarske (Executive Directors of Community Health Services and Psychiatric Services respectively). The task force members were senior administrators of the two branches, Joe Dvernichuk, Boris Titus and Evelyn Kent with Rick Roger Executive Director of Policy Research and Management Services acting as Secretary to the group and included Terry Russell, senior author of the 1980 Review as Special Advisor.

The Task Force was given "overall responsibility for the development of the child and youth health program." The task force was asked to develop detailed plans on improved integration of existing services and the implementation of new programs and services. The work of the task force was divided into two stages:

Stage I was to receive input on the report, consider organizational issues and confirm or modify the recommendations and initiate a review of program initiatives for 1981/82 and develop detailed plans for implementation by April 1, 1982.

Stage 2 tasks included developing the proposed organizational and management plan for Child and Youth Health Services, a 5 year program forecast including budgetary implications, an implementation plan for improvements to be made and the creation of working sub-groups as needed to deal with program specifics.

Much of the work of the task force was carried out by a

new entity, The Child and Youth Program Coordination Sub-committee made up of Marvin Klepsch, Abe Krahn, and Monica Hoffer representing Community Health and Tim Greenough, Zillah Parker and Laura Carment from Psychiatric Services. The subcommittee prepared a discussion paper outlining two options for discussion with staff and meetings involving the staff of the two branches and the Alcoholism Commission were held in regional centres across the province.

The first option left intact the two branches that were involved in children's health and added staff and programs.

- **Option 1** recommended the appointment of child and youth consultants in both Community Health and Psychiatric Services, provincial and regional coordinating committees and a reorganization within Psychiatric Services with the focus on the development of preventive outpatient programs and the establishment of a Child and Youth Division. Two sub-options were defined as well:

1.1 CHSB would establish "child and youth linkage workers in each of the ten health regions (Public health nurses whose responsibility would be to establish and maintain appropriate referral and triage mechanisms).

1.2 "Family Services" (not defined) be included in the new program mix.

- **Option 2** was a recommendation for major change in the configuration of the two involved branches. Option 2 was essentially as recommended in *Saskatchewan Health for Children and Youth* (the Russell Report) – the CHSB would assume responsibility for the community-based child and youth health services provided by PSB and the Alcoholism Commission.

The two options represent alternative means of improving

service delivery with the second option stressing a full integration of programs while the first option would increase coordinated program planning and development. Regional meetings were held to discuss the options. Comments on the two options were written by many of the Psychiatric Services regional staff. There were no joint regional submissions. Community Health and the Alcoholism Commission both provided summary responses prepared by their central offices.

The key findings of the Joint Task Force inquiry were that neither organizational option was unanimously endorsed at the regional level. All of the Community Health regions opted for the full integration of the programs albeit with varying levels of support. The Psychiatric Services regions were divided in their choice of option. The Alcoholism Commission opted for option 1.

The establishment of headquarters consultant positions in option one was generally viewed as a highly centralized and overly bureaucratic response to regional problems and further, as a diversion of resources from service delivery to administration. However, the reorganization within the Psychiatric Services Branch was accepted positively provided that such a reorganization would result in a legitimization of child and youth mental health services and the emergence of a mandate to develop community based preventive programming.

Those in the Psychiatric Services Branch who opposed the amalgamation of child and youth services in Community Health did so largely on the grounds that to do so would divide child and youth services from family services, especially in rural areas with few staff where the same staff members were providing services to both children and adults. Family services included: marriage counselling, family therapy, spousal battering and problems of the aged and elderly. Within Psychiatric Services, the transfer of services to Community Health was generally supported by child and youth workers, while "others, primarily psychiatrists, regional administrators, social workers and community health nurses, opposed this modification on the grounds that the consequences for the Psychiatric Services Branch would be dramatic."[139]

The Joint Task Force commented that there is a pervasive sense of lack of direction for the Psychiatric Services child and youth services resulting in ill-defined programs without a sense of purpose or mandate and thus significant regional variation in the provision of services. Further, Community Health staff lacks a clear understanding of the services provided by Psychiatric Services and the respective roles of the branches are unclear at the regional level.

The report of the Task Force states that both branches lack the necessary resources to adequately provide services for children and youth. While the regions cited numerous examples of coordination problems notably with case management, they expressed the view that the lack of adequate resources given the pool of unmet need in the community was more critical than problems in coordination. "It was asserted that allegations of inadequate coordination presumes the luxury of programs to synchronize. Conversely, coordination issues are frequently identified as key problems by external agencies such as school boards, community groups and consumers."[140]

In general, there was lukewarm support within Community Health for the amalgamation of child health services in all regions. Within Psychiatric Services there was strong support for the development of a strong health program for children and youth but little support for organizational change except from those who worked in Child and Youth Services. The outcome of the deliberations of the Joint Task Force was to recommend against the amalgamation of child, youth and family services under Community Health because it would have serious consequences for the Psychiatric Services Branch but to put forward a series of recommendations as alternatives to full amalgamation:

- Psychiatric Services should appoint a provincial Director of Child and Youth Services to coordinate program planning and development and to spearhead the process of legitimization of child and youth mental health services.

- Psychiatric Services should designate an identifiable child, youth and family service division and develop a service mandate.

- The Department of Health should establish a permanent Inter-Branch Coordinating Committee on Child and Youth Services to monitor program development, evaluate existing programs and clarify roles and responsibilities.

- The Department should implement a coterminous regional boundary structure for all programs as quickly as is feasible.

- Where compatible boundaries exist regional administrators should prepare a report identifying barriers to program coordination and the executive directors of each branch should jointly seek viable solutions to these problems.

- The branches should submit joint budget requests focused on child health.

- Community Health and Psychiatric Services should jointly develop policies regarding inter-branch sharing of client information that would permit access to client files by professionals in each branch.

- The Department should establish a Provincial Child and Youth Advisory Committee, comprising representatives from the organized treatment system, public and voluntary sectors, to advise the Department on the efficacy of existing programs/services and to assist in the development of a blueprint for the future.

- Administrators responsible for the school health demonstration project in Moose Jaw that had been recommended by the Review should ensure that Psychiatric

Services staff is involved in the delivery of service in the schools.

- A pilot project should be established in one region to test the efficacy of a joint Community Health- Psychiatric Services venture in service planning delivery. North Battleford region is preparing such a proposal.

The Joint Task Force Report was a reflection of the minimal consensus arrived at by the group and reflected general support for the status quo.

While changes to the Psychiatric Services Branch to formalize a Child and Youth Service were important steps, the Task Force and subsequently the Department did not address the importance of prevention and early intervention or the problems in coordination of community health services for children and youth.

With no structure or leadership in place following the report of the Task Force, the branches of the department most involved in providing community services to children and youth reverted to their historical positions and maintained their separate directions with little contact. Only the first two recommendations were acted upon and resulted in meaningful change to service delivery. Psychiatric Services did appoint a provincial Director of Child and Youth Services in 1982 and began the process of establishing an identifiable Child and Youth Mental Health Service in all regions.

What were the factors that blocked organizational change to improve services to children and youth?

The two branches had little history of working together on any common front. In the 1950s public health nurses had received training to enable them to provide follow-up care in the community for those discharged from mental hospitals. However this training had not been updated or maintained. By the 1960s Community Health was increasingly focused on preschool children. Their predominant business was prevention and early intervention. The availability of educational psychologists within Community Health was seen by staff of the branch as sufficient to provide follow-up as needed for youngsters with mental health problems. Within the Psychiatric Services Branch the focus on service delivery had moved from mental hospitals to community psychiatry however the client group remained the chronically mentally ill adult. The training program for psychiatric nurses was a major thrust that improved the care of the chronically mentally ill. However, there were unresolved issues between the registered nurses and the newer profession of registered psychiatric nurses which resulted in public health nurses and psychiatric nurses having difficulty working together. All of these factors served to ensure that the branches had little in common and little likelihood of making a smooth transition to one management.

Evelyn Kent, Associate Executive Director of Community Health who had recently arrived in Saskatchewan and so was unaware and uninvolved in the history between the two branches in her summary of the eight regional meetings stated:

> "There is little understanding of roles and functions between professional staffs in the two Branches. It was very profitable for both branches to have these joint regional meetings so that the lack of knowledge of each other and in some cases, open hostilities (which I believe have mainly historic basis – and can be addressed more sanely with our present staff) were aired and in most cases reason prevailed at the conclusion of each meeting." And further: "I was amazed to hear that bureaucratic organizational models were perceived by field staff to create insurmountable obstacles that severely cripple the flow of information. ... Our two branches are perceived as separate "agencies" and therefore information belongs to one and not the other. In fact cannot be shared with the other!"[141]

It is little wonder that the two branches had difficulty in considering organizational proposals that affected them both. Within Psychiatric Services in the 1960s and early 1970s there was an ongoing problem among the professions providing service, each jockeying for power within the system that was developing. This has been well described by Harley Dickinson.[142] It is also referenced in Chapter 6.

Psychiatry was predominant and all of the regional executive directors were psychiatrists and their primary responsibility was treating people with chronic mental illness. Psychiatric nurses and social workers vied with one another for supremacy within the developing outpatient system. There were few psychologists available. The system was based on a professional department model and all were uneasy with the interdisciplinary approach that was being taken in the beginnings of the development of Child and Youth Services.

An organizational structure based on a professional discipline model was a major factor in the response of the Psychiatric Services staff and administration to the recommendations for organizational change that would develop a child health service.

Loss of staff was the other major factor in discussions about the possible transfer of child and youth services from Psychiatric Services. Many regions had not yet identified staff dedicated to providing services to young clients. Instead staff members would each be assigned a percentage of time for this purpose along with other duties. Up to 1979, there was no clear mandate to provide specialized mental health services for children and youth and thus the service was developing in many different ways in different regions. Certainly, there was no priority given to services to young clients in most regions. From the perspective of Community Health Services Branch there was no program to transfer, rather it was an undefined set of program activities with no mandate and no policy formulation.

The outcome of the regional discussions was to maintain the status quo. Psychiatric Services did not wish to give up child and youth services. It was a vital and growing part of their services. Community Health wished to continue to develop preventive and early childhood services and was not willing to take responsibility for a multi-disciplinary targeted treatment program. While everyone agreed that more coordination at the planning and service delivery levels was needed, with no new structural mechanism to encourage it, coordination remained a sometimes thing, dependent upon personal relationships rather than expectation or department policy.

The only bright light arising from the Task Force deliberations was the decision by Psychiatric Services to appoint a Director of Child and Youth Services and to begin to work towards a viable program.

THE INTERNATIONAL YEAR OF YOUTH IN SASKATCHEWAN

For a description of national initiatives during the IYY, see chapter 2.

In 1985 the United Nations honoured youth with an International Year. The most tangible IYC activity sponsored by the Department of Health in Saskatchewan was part of a demonstration project – Health Promotion and Counselling for Youth – housed at Regina Child and Youth Services during the development phases. The project was jointly funded by Saskatchewan Health along with the Family Planning Division and the Health Promotion Directorate of Health Canada.

Three *Activity Learning Guides* were published for youth group leaders and teachers. The guides were written to encourage health learning opportunities for youth in schools and community organizations.

The first guide, *Communication Skills for Youth*,[143] focused on developing leadership skills through active, experiential learning to develop positive peer interaction in developing communication and leadership skills. *Food Fitness and Feelings*[144] provided the teacher or youth group leader with an exciting range of learning activities geared to younger teens who are concerned with the issues of self-image, peer pressure, the importance of nutrition and fitness. *Discovering You*[145] was the theme for the third *Activity Learning Guide*.

As well as researching the materials and developing the *Activity Learning Guides* the project developed and piloted a series of youth health conferences that involved young people, teachers and health and social service workers in the community. The focus of the conferences was to encourage youth to develop Youth Health Councils in the community or the schools. The new youth organizations that developed were served by a Keeping in Touch Newsletter – "Health is it!" The Youth Health Councils developed health action plans for themselves and their communities. Health topics varied from alcohol and drug education to fitness breaks at school and school lunch programs operated by the students in home economics classes.

In one small community the students could not get permission to have a suicide prevention seminar in the school because of administration's fear of the topic. Undeterred, they organized a weekend seminar in a community hall that was the best-attended event of the year. The youth led Health Councils whether based in the schools or the community provided a much needed opportunity for youth to take action on behalf of their own health.

8

The Great Leap Forward in the 1980s

GETTING READY TO MAKE THE LEAP

L arge organizations do not change easily or quickly. We have already noted when discussing the development of mental hospitals early in the century and the later move to empty those hospitals and focus on community psychiatry that change happens most quickly and effectively when three factors are in place. The three factors that underlie government change are political commitment, enthusiastic and committed professional leadership and the support of community advocates. Child and Youth Mental Health Services in Saskatchewan did not have political commitment or community advocacy on its side. Many community members had worked enthusiastically on the cause that mattered to them personally (see Chapter 5 for a description of several of the child-serving private organizations that had been created by groups of concerned parents). However few were sufficiently interested in the overall provision of a comprehensive mental health program for children and youth to advocate for such a program.

From the early 1960s on there had been many attempts to focus attention on the needs of children and youth with mental health problems. However, the attention of the politicians was never captured nor were members of the general public involved in advocacy on behalf of the development of services.

Prominent among the many reports which pointed out the service gaps and suggested solutions was the 1964 report of the Interdepartmental Coordinating Committee on Rehabilitation – *Services to Emotionally Disturbed Children in Saskatchewan.*[146] It was published just as a new Liberal government headed by Ross Thatcher came to power in the province. The timing could not have been worse as the Liberals were committed to smaller government not to increased programs.

Asselstine's Three Year Development Plan for Service to Children and Adolescents[147] had been quickly shelved although some new staff had been added to the eight regional offices as part of the institutional downsizing exercise.

The Health Thrust Committee Report[148] by Treherne, Russell and Kelly while mainly focused on identifying problems in the children's services system, had recommended the creation of provincial planning mechanisms for an overall mental health system for children and youth. However, the government of the day chose to implement three costly but important new programs – a dental plan for children, a prescription drug plan and a program to provide aids to independent living for people with handicaps.

Russell's 1974 planning report[149] and the establishment of the Provincial Child and Youth Advisory Committee in 1978 were useful activities that provided focus within the Psychiatric Services Branch and helped to strengthen the program internally but did not involve either the politicians or the public.

In 1979, the International Year of the Child, the Review of Child Health Services created a plan to amalgamate all community child health services under one administration (See chapter 7). However, the bureaucracies involved were unwilling to support this move to establish a community child health service as they feared the loss of individual power even though each was unable to make a priority for children's services within their own mandate.

However, ultimately deliberations in the health department about the consolidation of child health services resulted in the Psychiatric Services Branch committing to develop a provincial Child and Youth Mental Health Service. The branch agreed to establish the position of provincial director to oversee policy and program development, to hire regional directors responsible for program operations and to submit a treasury board request for new money to support the new program.

1981 PROVINCIAL PROGRAM OVERVIEW

In June of 1981 Terry Russell prepared a Provincial Program Overview to summarize the issues facing the Child and Youth Mental Health Program in the province.[150] The paper was developed as the starting point for the Psychiatric Services Branch to put forward Treasury Board proposals on behalf of child and youth mental health services for the 1982-83 fiscal year.

The Department of Health was still following through with the recommendations of the Joint Task Force on Health Services for Children and Youth. The task force had recommended joint budget submissions. The joint submission consisted of each Branch (Psychiatric Services and Community Health) making a submission and the two submissions were stapled together for presentation to the Minister and eventually Treasury Board. The branches were still not working closely together.

The Psychiatric Services Branch paper[151] began with a problem statement that was summarized as follows:

"Specific problems that have impeded the development of a province-wide community mental health program for children and youth include

- lack of priority, unclear mandate,

- no administrative program development structure,

- PSB historical focus upon hospital-based psychiatric care and follow-up services for adults,

- general budget restraint on labour intensive human services."

The discussion paper went on to describe the magnitude of the problem, it outlined issues involving youth lifestyle choices, current service utilization and the problems of service planning and delivery coordination and identified five strategies for developing a child and youth mental health service.

Youth, Health and Lfestyles[152] had found in their survey of young people that youth perceived a lack of accessible and responsive counselling services for health and social concerns. It is only in a crisis that young people look for solutions to lifestyle problems. The survey found that peers were the major sources of information about lifestyle problems and provided the greatest support in times of trouble.

The overview paper outlined problems in horizontal and vertical integration of services including the lack of provincial policy and planning and the resulting variations in regional service provision that confused consumers and other agencies.

The provincial program overview focused on the development of a mental health service for children and youth and provided five strategies for planning and development of the new service system. The strategies pulled together the current status of service delivery and added innovations that were being developed in the regions or that were seen as highest priority.

Strategy 1 – Increased Service Capacity and Improved Distribution of Resources.

- Appoint a provincial director responsible for planning and provincial standards,

- Appoint full time regional directors of CYMHS,

- Set minimum staffing standards at one person year per 10,000 population under 19,

- Make regional boundaries coterminous,

- Establish district offices within regions,

- Develop training for and employ local community mental health workers in small communities,

- Develop a volunteer program to provide supports in rural communities,

- Provide consulting services to northern Saskatchewan from North Battleford and Prince Albert, and

- Develop formal consulting relationships with specialized agencies such as Alvin Buchwald Centre, Wascana Hospital, Ranch Ehrlo, and Child and Youth Psychiatry.

Strategy 2 – Consultation and Linkage

- Regional directors will develop links with CHSB including managerial coordination meetings, referral and case coordination mechanisms, information and joint record sharing and joint program development.

- Provide staff for regional pilot project development: North Battleford (Joint PSB/CHSB Service Coordination), Moose Jaw (School-based Health Project), and Rosetown (Wheatlands Project).

- Establish a Family Therapy Training and Consultation Unit at MacNeill Clinic in Saskatoon.

- Hire a pediatrics psychology consultant in Regina where there are no hospital psychology departments.

- Regina Region will develop consultation models: long term planning for children in the care of the Minister of Social Services; court and community programs for delinquent youth; community-based family service programs; and programs for infants and young children.

Strategy 3 – Special Target Programs for Mental Health Education.

- Two target groups for community mental health education were identified: parent education and peer counseling for youth.

- A grant of $45,000 be made to the Regina Parent Education Association to further develop the voluntary program in place for six years.

- Hire a central office mental health education consultant to develop parent education resources in concert with the community colleges and provide in-service education to staff.

- A federal research grant of $100,000 per year for three years has been received to develop specialized counselling and educational resources for high risk youth and nine new positions are requested to develop and monitor regional programs to be developed in conjunction with the research.

- A peer counselling pilot project is planned for the Regina region.

- $80,000 is requested for provincial public education and information regarding the new program for the mental health of children and youth.

Strategy 4 – Special Target Program for Difficult to Manage Youth

- An in-home support worker in North Battleford, a

home-based early intervention family support program in Regina and a community recreation program in Saskatoon were planned.

- A three year pilot program in Regina to provide family support services following emergency ward care for children and youth following suicide attempts and serious injury.

- A specialized residential treatment program for older youth (15 to 22) with severe emotional problems often associated with other issues such as borderline intelligence or delinquency would be established by Ranch Ehrlo.

Strategy 5 – Special Target Progam for Natives

- $320,000 was requested to provide grants to native organizations to hire native family support workers to work closely with Child and Youth Mental Health offices in the regions.

- A community development worker was requested for North Battleford to develop a community day program for youth.

- One staff member to be hired in each of Regina and Saskatoon to provide training opportunities and monitor the new native program initiatives.

The strategies in the discussion paper all built on and were derived from existing initiatives and were in harmony with identified regional priorities. The primary purpose of the paper was to outline a range of initiatives that could comprise a viable community mental health program for children and youth in Saskatchewan. The broad range of proposals had been generated within the PSB during 1981. Priorities were not established, rather the approach taken was to provide a menu of possibilities from which the Department of Health might choose and which in the future might serve to define the program as it developed.

On the basis of the discussion paper a budget request for just over one million dollars was developed. It would have supported hiring an additional 39 mental health workers. As a matter of historical interest, the following represents the staffing by region and by discipline at the end of March 1982.

At the time there were 51.4 person years of professional staff providing services to children and youth in the province. The total number of full and part time staff involved was 70.

PROFESSIONAL STAFFING BY REGION IN MARCH 1982

	Person Years	Part Time Staff	Full Time Staff
Prince Albert	4	8 PT	0
North Battleford	4.2	5 PT	0
Swift Current	2.7	9 PT	0
Moose Jaw	2.1	7 PT	0
Weyburn	3.5	4 PT	0
Regina	19	0	19
Yorkton	1.8	3 PT	0
Saskatoon	14	0	14

TOTAL STAFFING BY JOB CLASSIFICATION MARCH 1982

	Person Years
Child Psychiatrist	2.3
Psychiatrist	5
Psychologist	21.0
Social Worker	18.83

CMH Nurse	.88
Speech Therapist	2.0
Adjunctive Therapist	5.9
Clerical Support staff	8.6
Total staff	**60**

The discussion paper and the Psychiatric Services Branch B Budget Request for 1982-83 were discussed at a meeting on April 6/7, 1982 called at the request of David Kelly, Associate Deputy Minister to discuss future directions in child and youth services in the Psychiatric Services Branch.

THE GREAT LEAP FORWARD

The 1982-83 B Budget Request[153] is the document that legitimizes a Child and Youth Mental Health Service in Saskatchewan. Acceptance of this document by Treasury Board provided for the following, all of which were recommended by the Joint Task Force:

- Establishment of a clear mandate for PSB to provide mental health services to children and youth.

- Establish the position of provincial Director of Child and Youth Services.

- Consolidate existing mental health services for children and youth in each region.

- Increase the service capacity and improve the distribution of resources throughout the province.

- Improve consultation services and coordination with Community Health Services and other agencies as necessary.

Treasury Board initially approved a budget increase sufficient to provide a salary for the Provincial Director and increased service capacity of four new positions in each of Moose Jaw, Swift Current, Prince Albert and Yorkton. Similar increases of staff in Weyburn and North Battleford were to be made by using existing positions. However, following further review and reduction in the total 1982-83 Health Department budget the number of new positions was reduced to 9. The final budget approval of 9 new and eight transfer positions was considerably less than the branch request for 39 new positions. Nevertheless, the injection of new staff went a long way towards developing service capacity across the province.

The provincial budget of 1982 marked the "great leap forward" for Child and Youth Mental Health Services. The branch received a clear mandate to provide services. A new provincial director, Laura Carment was hired to organize, plan and develop the services. Existing service capacity was consolidated and improved with new resources. A directional message was given to the new service – "Improve consultation services and coordination with Community Health Services and other agencies." One can truly say that the new program of community mental health services for children and youth was born during the budget debate of 1982-83.

For many years services in the regions had depended upon the interest of one or more of the staff. Availability of service waxed and waned as staff came and went. There was no overall commitment to the development of a program for children and youth provincially or in the regions. This began to change with the budget of 1982-83 which brought new staff positions for the outlying regions and most importantly which spelled out for the Psychiatric Services Branch the mandate to proceed with the development of mental health services for children and youth.

CMHA TASK FORCE

During this same time period, the Canadian Mental Health Association organized a task force committee on Mental Health Services in Saskatchewan chaired by Ian MacDonald, professor of psychiatry at the University of Saskatchewan. Their report, a wide-ranging document titled, *the Forgotten Constituents*, was released in May 1983 . The section on children and youth is introduced with the statement:

> "The mental health problems of children and adolescents many be defined from many points of view, including the parent, the educator, the police and courts, social workers, physicians, psychiatrists and clinical psychologists." [154]

It is surprising that the report does not include children and youth themselves as defining their mental health problems as the report was published just before the International Year of Youth. The report reflects the varied input of task force members by providing a series of recommendations that while important in themselves are not based in a coherent analysis. Rather the report focuses on a wide range of improvements that might be made to the overall system.

Recommendations included:

- a request for money to provide a Directory of Services;

- demonstration projects to determine effective and efficient methods of providing rural services;

- immediate implementation of family support measures included in the Family Services Act of 1973;

- implementation of the Law Reform Commission recommendation on age of consent to be considered the age of understanding;

- equitable foster home rates;

- intensive summer recreation programs;

- increased funds from the Department of Education for personal counselling and mental health consultation;

- funding by the Department of Education for the development of a high cost funding category for emotionally disturbed children and additional funds for low cost students;

- preventive education programs for suicide and teen pregnancy; and

- funds be provided to CMHA for four rural demonstration projects to develop voluntary mental health action groups.

The report also recognizes the need for and recommends increased special services for high risk hospitalized children and psychiatric patients, calls for early screening and early diagnosis of mental health problems and lastly, the development of a full range of diagnostic and residential mental health treatment programs in each region.

The report provided an expensive menu of recommendations but it was not seen by government as a platform for change. The preparation of MacDonald's report was supported by the Canadian Mental Health Association, however, there was little public comment at the time of its release and no concerted follow-up or advocacy for change associated with it.

During the years from 1982 through to 1986 there was gradual growth in the provincial mental health program for children and youth. The provincial director established regular meetings of the regional directors. Provincial level policy was developed and the groundwork for on-going development was established. Five new positions to provide specialized mental health services to comply with the new federal Young Offenders Act were allocated in the 1984-85 budget and another four were added to address the needs of young sexual offenders by the end of the decade. The new program of Child and Youth Mental Health Services was fast becoming a vibrant component of the provincial program of mental health services.

9

Common Themes Revisited 1985 and Onward

NATIONAL INITIATIVES

The last fifteen years of the twentieth century was an active and productive era for children's mental health at the national level. It was also the period when the provinces and the Government of Canada first established a formal mechanism for those who worked with children and youth to meet, share information and to develop a national perspective.

At the beginning of this time period, in most provinces the administrative responsibility for mental health services for children and youth was lodged with the management structure in the Department of Health that was responsible for adult mental health services. As a consequence, those serving children competed for policy attention and resources with a much larger and more powerful sector. This was changing in a number of jurisdictions and as well as describing new national policy initiatives this chapter describes and compares the various management structures and service delivery priorities of the provinces.

In April of 1986 the Federal/Provincial/Territorial Advisory

Committee on Mental Health established a Working Group on the Mental Health of Children and Youth. The advisory committee members were the people responsible for children's mental health services in their jurisdiction. The Working Group was the first national body focused on the mental health of children and youth and it was established with the following objectives:

- to provide advice on mental health policy designed to address conditions of psychiatric distress, disorder and disability in children and youth;

- to assist in the development of program and resource material for mental health workers, policy makers and program directors; and

- to provide opportunities at the national level for information exchange.

The establishment of the Working Group was an important recognition of the fact that to best serve children and youth, mental health policy and resource development is different from that needed for adults. The opportunity to meet with colleagues at a national table and share solutions to common problems was an important step in the growth of the program across the country.

An early publication of the Working Group, *Foundations for the Future*[155] describes the history, philosophy of services, current status and recommends building blocks for the future. For the first time in Canada there was a document that described the mental health needs of young people and the approaches taken in Canada to meet those needs.

The priority issues for the Working Group included planning and coordination of a broadly-based children's services network, the integration of hospital and community mental health systems and planning to develop preventive and early intervention services. An over-arching priority was the need to address the immediacy of service needs for the young.

In preparing the foundation document, the Working Group identified a number of areas of priority concern and commissioned papers from Canadian experts.

The titles and authors are included for those who may wish to follow up on the areas of priority identified by the Working Group:

- Ingredients Towards a Philosophy of Service Delivery to Children (Cyr, 1988);

- Suicide Prevention for the Young (Dyck, 1988);

- Mental Health Status of Children in Canada (Krzanowska, 1988);

- Promoting the Mental Health of Children and Youth: A Critical Review of the Literature (Ledingham and Crombie, 1987);

- Funding Issues in Children's Mental Health (McLellan, 1988);

- Ranges of Rates of Prevalence of Childhood Mental Illness (Renney, 1988);

- Substance Abuse by Children and Youth (Turanski, 1988);

- Mental Health Legislation for Children and Youth in Canada (Russell and Sigmundson, 1988); and,

- Research Priorities for Children's Mental Health (Thompson, 1988).

Foundations for the Future is the most important source of information for those interested in the mental health of children and youth in Canada. It describes with great clarity the history and current status of services up to 1990 and provides direction for the future.

In the early 1990s a reorganization within Health Canada brought to the Working Group a new name --Federal/ Provincial/Territorial Working Group on the Mental Health of Children and Youth – and a new home in the Childhood and Youth Division of the Population Health branch of Health Canada. The Committee was now distanced from the formal mental health system represented at the national level by the Advisory Committee on Mental Health.

The committee, in its new home, continued to work on its primary concern, the mental health of children and youth with an emphasis on service delivery. There was always a tension between the pressures on the federal representatives to focus on changing federal priorities and the desire of the provincial representatives to emphasize service delivery. The group was responsible for two planning papers, *A Self Regulating Service Delivery System for Children and Youth At Risk*[156] compiled by Wade Junek and Gus Thompson and *Moving Towards Best Practices*, a project led by Joe Kluger that was never completed.

However, the priority of the federal division was moving towards early childhood, nutrition and Aboriginal health. With constant reorganizations, staffing problems and increasing budget constraints at the federal level and an unwillingness of the provinces to share the cost of committee expenses, the committee quietly folded around the turn of the century. Members continued to share information but without regular contact in meetings there was little focus or creative spark.

INTER-PROVINCIAL COMPARISONS OF SERVICE DELIVERY MANAGEMENT

During this time period there were three national surveys on child and youth mental health provision in the provinces and territories. The following material is summarized from the three surveys – Doherty[157] on behalf of the Government of Alberta, Campbell and Thompson[158] on behalf of the Federal/ Provincial Working Group on the Mental Health of Children and Youth, and Russell[159] on behalf of the Childhood and Youth Division, Population Health Branch of Health Canada.

All three projects used essentially the same approach. In each case, the survey document was completed by the provincial department or ministry responsible for mental health services for children and youth. The surveys are comparable in that for the most part they built on the preceding survey and thus covered common ground although with slightly different emphases.

Of particular emphasis in the Doherty document were four issues identified by the Government of Alberta – the development of a continuum of services, quality control, rural service provision and services to native children and families. Because there is often overlap between child welfare and mental health systems concerning the provision of services to children and youth with emotional and behavioural problems the services provided by child welfare have also been considered.

Government officials in most provinces indicated that neglected and abused children are primarily the responsibility of child welfare and youngsters who are psychotic or severely depressed are primarily the responsibility of mental health services. However, there was little consensus within or among the provinces regarding the appropriate locus of responsibility for those with behavioural or emotional problems and generally, both systems provide services to children with emotional and behavioural problems. As a result of this uncertainty of responsibility, Doherty paid special attention to the relationships between the two systems.

In summarizing the results of the 1985 survey, Doherty notes that in all provinces except Ontario, mental health services for children and youth are provided by the same government department and administration as are mental health services for adults. Child welfare services are generally under the jurisdiction of a separate department. Six of the ten provinces, provide the majority of mental health services to youngsters through a network of child/adult outpatient clinics supplemented by psychiatric units in general hospitals.

All provinces have a Mental Health Act that governs the provision of services and is primarily focused on inpatient care. Ontario also has a Children's Mental Health Centre Act 1968-69, governing the establishment, funding, licensing and standard setting for children's mental health centres. By regulation under the Ontario Act, the facilities are also designated psychiatric facilities under the Mental Health Act. The mental health centres range from inpatient and residential facilities to community mental health clinics.

Alberta's Child Welfare Service has developed secure custody legislation that allows a special designation by a psychiatrist or psychologist to be made on behalf of emotionally disturbed youth that allows them to be placed and held involuntarily in residential custody to protect them while an assessment is completed. British Columbia has passed similar legislation but has not proclaimed it. In both provinces the legislation is similar to mental health legislation but operated outside of the formal mental health system.

All provinces have child welfare legislation that allows for services to be provided on a voluntary basis and the vast majority of residential services (foster, group homes and child care institutions) and many family support services are provided by the child welfare system. At this time Saskatchewan had a six bed psychiatric unit at University Hospital and a six bed group home in Saskatoon funded by the Ministry of Health and operated under the Mental Health Act. Hospital inpatient units in each region routinely admitted older youth as needed and often made placements in approved adult boarding homes.

Most provinces have designated the Ministry of Education to provide services for children with emotional and behavioural problems and this is formalized in legislation governing schools in Saskatchewan, British Columbia and Ontario.

The core child and youth mental health services that are provided across the country are summarized by Doherty as:

- Provision of in-depth assessment that provides an understanding of the factors internal to the child and external factors in the environment that are contributing to the problem behaviour;

- Determination of the intervention most likely to address the child's needs and development of an intervention plan;

- Case consultation to those implementing the plan; and

- Provision of highly specialized and/or more intensive interventions.

With this core of services and in cooperation with the child welfare authorities it is intended that the mental health needs of youngsters will be met.

The Saskatchewan program provided all four of these core services through a network of eight regional mental health centres. However, only British Columbia, Manitoba and New Brunswick had formalized coordination mechanisms at the local level. Similarly, most provinces did not have formal inter-departmental planning and coordination committees responsible for services to youngsters. Rather planning coordination among responsible departments tended to depend upon ad hoc and time-limited task forces to address specific issues.

In Saskatchewan at the time, rural services were provided from the eight regional centres and staffing was not sufficient to develop satellite clinics. Several of the regions -- Swift Current, North Battleford, Prince Albert and Weyburn were beginning to establish regular traveling clinics. The Doherty report indicates that while there were no specialized mental health services for aboriginal people in Saskatchewan, formalized consulting arrangements existed between mental health and aboriginal service delivery organizations, for example, in Regina with Peyakowak and a youth group home. These agencies were funded by the social services department and were administered, operated and staffed by natives.

In 1988 an update of the Doherty report prepared by Thompson and Campbell outlines the minor administrative and program changes that had taken place since the publication of the 1985 report. They summarize the changes by stating:

"Small changes have been made to the children's mental health system throughout the country, however, the children's system is still seen as under resourced. Many of the changes that have occurred have been made to the adult mental health system with minor benefits trickling down to the children's systems. Administrative changes appear to have been more prevalent and these may improve linkages and reduce fragmentation."[160]

The administrative changes mostly had to do with moving government branches between departments and thus reorganizing the linkages. Such reorganizations did not take place in Saskatchewan at this time.

The Russell[161] document provides a more detailed inventory of children's services in eight of the 12 provinces and territories that existed in the latter part of the nineties. For a variety of reasons four jurisdictions including Saskatchewan, did not respond to the survey request. However, in the intervening years there had been no major program changes in Saskatchewan's mental health program for children and youth. It remained a responsibility of the Department of Health and was delivered in conjunction with the Mental Health Regional programs. In describing the results of the 2000 survey, comments about Saskatchewan will be inserted in order to show the developments in this province.

As well as surveying the mental health services for children and youth and child welfare services the Russell report outlines the hospital-based and residential services, medical services, preventive and early intervention services, alcohol and drug services, young offender services, rehabilitation, child care, and education. A very complete picture of service organization and delivery is provided. Each province and territory has its own unique organizational structure. However, there were several common themes evident in the provincial submissions:

- There was a general move to more integrated and less complex structures with more services for children and youth under a single management authority.

- There was increased independence or autonomy for operating regions, especially in the health sector.

- Coordinating or integrating structures for planning and policy development across structures were becoming common

- The differences in funding structures impede service delivery, for example, physicians (fee for service), schools and health districts/regions (global funding), and community services (operate as government funded and managed agencies).

- Systems with regional boards of governance, for example, schools and health districts/regions tend to be more stable.

- The child protection field continues as a high priority because of media coverage that is highly critical of the handling of high profile cases.

- A highly organized advocacy body in a sector, especially of parents, leads to stability of funding and organization.

- Policy and service delivery directions continue to change focus and balance based on the relative priority given to one or more of the following principles: supporting families, increasing parental independence, encouraging child development and ensuring child protection.

COMMON THEMES

Throughout the decade of the nineties the problems of coordination for planning and delivering services at the provincial, regional and local levels had become a major issue uppermost in the minds of everyone who responded to the survey. The three largest provinces and the smallest had created integrated departments or ministries with responsibility for a wide range of services to children and youth. Newfoundland and Labrador and Nunavut had already integrated Community Health and Social Services in a similar approach. The remaining provinces (including Saskatchewan) had introduced coordinating mechanisms for planning at the central level to ensure that services were working together.

At the local level there were a variety of approaches to ensure that services worked together and were coordinated for individual youngsters as needed. The most sophisticated approach to local service delivery coordination was in British Columbia which has had a series of local Child and Youth Committees across the province since the 1970s. As well, BC has developed an integrated case management approach and provided training province-wide to staff of all child-serving organizations. More recently, in 1997, BC created a new ministry – the Ministry for Children and Families (now renamed the Ministry of Children and Family Development) -- bringing together child welfare, public health, human services, mental health, youth justice, alcohol and drug programs and services for people with developmental disabilities. It must be noted that the BC integrated ministry has reorganized again. The public health and alcohol and drug programs have been returned to the Ministry of Health and are now administered through the five regional health boards. At the time of writing another reorganization is planned.

A second major theme that developed in the responses to the survey was the need to take a population health approach in the development of health and social programs to take into account such factors as employment and environmental factors and educational levels in the community. The population health approach has many proponents but there was little effective change seen on the basis of the survey responses. Time will tell if this approach will begin to affect the planning and delivery of services in a significant manner.

Health promotion and early intervention, concepts that

have been around for a long time, were described as a primary focus in many provinces. Well known programs such as Nobody's Perfect, HeadStart and several well baby programs were identified as present in the service system. Federal government leadership and especially funding was central to the development of these approaches and there was concern raised about their continuation should the funding stop.

The last theme that was on the minds of those in most jurisdictions was that of evaluation and the development of outcome measures. However, there was little specific information in the survey responses to show how the issue of evaluation was being addressed. The Russell report comments:

> "It is usual for health and social programs to change slowly, often driven by political agenda and with little formal use of program evaluation. It is also usual for rhetoric about change to precede change. Consequently, we may see the beginning of an approach to program development that is based in program evaluation."[162]

Whether or not there has been an increase in program evaluation in the years since the last survey is not known. One can only hope that there is more than rhetoric about evaluation and that those involved in planning and providing services are indeed working towards a better system in a formalized manner basing the changes on sound evaluation, research and evidence-based practice.

It is important to note that there is no provincial or national non-governmental body whose mandate is to advocate on behalf of youngsters with mental health problems or for the improvement in services on their behalf. Those organizations that exist tend to be time-limited and focused on a specific issue or concern or they are focused on a specific type of problem, for example, autism and related disorders. The public advocacy focus on the mental health of children and youth is mostly limited to groups of professionals working together on behalf of those that they serve. Professionals are often frustrated when they attempt to plan beyond the specifics of their own work or on behalf of individual youngsters. It is interesting to speculate about the impact that might be made by a broadly based public advocacy group concerned with the mental health needs of children and youth. Such groups, especially those that are parent-dominated, have had a remarkable impact on services for those with learning and developmental disabilities and autism and related disorders.

In summary, the programs of child and youth mental health services across the country have not changed substantially since the original national survey in 1985.

The management structure in Saskatchewan remains similar to that of most provinces. It is funded by the Department of Health and operated regionally as a component of a mental health service that is predominantly concerned with the needs of adults with severe and chronic mental illness. The major change is that the regional mental health programs are now managed by regional authorities along with all other health funded services. Mental health services are no longer administered directly by the Department of Health.

10
Moving Ahead

FADS AND FASHIONS

Looking at the past twenty-five years, certain common trends have been evident in most if not all provinces. Organizational initiatives and illnesses or conditions that have attracted major media attention have shaped service delivery in Saskatchewan and elsewhere. These fashions have popped up at different times in different provinces and territories but have tended to be common experiences in all jurisdictions. Frequently the federal government has been responsible for planning and funding new initiatives which often become part of provincial programs because of the funding incentive offered.

One could call these trends or activities fads and fashions. Each tends to develop independently often following the publication of research or committee reports on specific issues or as a media issue. The fads are not the result of a comprehensive review of the needs of youngsters rather they are usually more narrowly focused. As well, it is most usual for them to develop across the usual jurisdictional or service management mandates and boundaries.

FUNDING FADS

In recent years a number of conditions related to the mental health of children and youth have captured media and public interest and thus political support. The outcome has been the development of specialized programs to meet specific needs. In Saskatchewan, Child and Youth Mental Health Services has been quick to respond to special initiatives and thus the programs offered have become differentiated to meet the newly identified needs. However, at the same time there has been no professional leadership, political commitment or public advocacy directed at meeting the broader mental health needs of youngsters in Saskatchewan during this time.

New funding has been provided to address youth suicide, young sexual offenders, youth at risk of offending, the needs of First Nations families, early childhood intervention, coordinated behaviour management, and autism treatment. From 1992 to 2004 funding for these initiatives has more than doubled the available staff in the provincial program through an increase of 63.5 positions. Responding to special needs that are largely defined by others might be called entrepreneurial program development. It has increased services available in specific areas of responsibility. The entrepreneurial model shifts the focus of clinical efforts in the directions specified by the new funding but does not necessarily result in an increase in the overall capacity to meet the mental health needs of the children. As they say in the movies, follow the money. That's where you'll find the services.

MEDIA FOCUS ON CHILD PROTECTION CASES

From time to time a child dies at the hand of parents or other caregivers and this tragic event sometimes receives massive media attention. The same has been true when dramatic sexual abuse cases receive much public attention. This has occurred in several provinces in recent years. The resulting self-examination by the organizations involved can and has in several provinces resulted in a complete reorganization of the delivery of social and mental health services to children. When the reorganization is driven primarily by the notion of preventing abuse and neglect it has not always resulted in an organizational structure best designed to meet the mental health needs of children and youth.

REORGANIZING GOVERNMENT DOWNSIZING

During the 1980s initiatives to downsize the civil service were fashionable. All provinces in Canada have experimented with initiatives to downsize government always as cost-saving measures and often involving rhetoric about privatization, a measure that is deemed by its proponents to be more efficient and thus less costly overall. In Saskatchewan early in their second term the Conservative government of Grant Devine introduced many initiatives to downsize government.

In 1987 the government instituted two measures in parallel that had a significant negative effect on mental health services. Firstly, vacant staff positions were deleted and secondly, an early retirement program was instituted and the positions of those who retired were deleted.

Overall the Mental Health Services Branch lost approximately 100 staff positions and the impact on Child and Youth Mental Health was considerable. As described in Chapter 8 the increase of staff from 1982 to 1986 was thirteen positions or 25%. In 1987 seven of the thirteen new positions were clawed back through the Devine government's downsizing initiative.

Laura Carment (1988) the provincial director of Child and Youth Mental Health commented on the impact of downsizing.

> "In summary, most of the gains made between 1982 and 1986 have been reversed. Resources for serving children and youth remain uneven across the province, with rural areas lacking continuity in the provision of basic services and urban centres facing inadequate access due to insufficient resources in relation to complex needs."[163]

This was a great blow to the new service for children and youth. Similar events have occurred in other provinces. And as provincial economies improved and governments changed, staff numbers increased and programs were reintroduced or expanded. However the children and families who spent too long on wait lists or who never did receive services because of downsizing exercises may live with the consequences of this for the rest of their lives.

REGIONALIZATION OF HEALTH SERVICES

In Saskatchewan as in other provinces, there has been a move to the establishment of regional health authorities that are responsible for the administration of all provincially funded health services. Prior to this, health administration was governed by a hodgepodge of mechanisms. Elected district boards were responsible for hospitals, an appointed provincial commission oversaw alcohol and drug services, appointed regional boards managed public health, and mental health and continuing care for the elderly were administered directly by the Department of Health. Regional boundaries were not coterminous and overall planning was almost impossible.

Starting in 1992, Saskatchewan moved towards a regional system of administration for all health services by establishing 32 health districts. An early result was the consolidation of hospital services and the closure of a number of small hospitals. The initial focus of the district boards was on acute and continuing care and ambulance services.

Subsequently, in 1995 the Department of Health devolved responsibility for management of all health-funded programs to the regional boards. Up to this time, many of the community programs such as mental health services were administered directly by the Department of Health. The Regina-Qu'Appelle Region took over the management of all health-funded services. Mental health and addiction services were amalgamated under a single manager. The opportunities for these two organizations to work together were thus improved greatly as were the possibilities of working more closely with all other health services.

However, those working in mental health, public health and alcohol and drug services were troubled by their loss of priority and access to government decision-making.

Additionally one result of regionalization was the loss of central office administration and associated power and thus no policy and planning direction or protection for smaller programs that were not involved in acute or continuing care. The loss of policy and planning direction remains an issue that requires attention. Working together in partnership with education, child welfare and youth corrections at the local and regional levels demands a provincial planning and policy framework that is coherent and provides visible leadership.

The loss of a strong voice in central government concerned with and advocating on behalf of the mental health needs of children and youth leaves a gap in the development of policy and planning for evidence-based practice. Further, the system is without a capacity to monitor quality and ensure equality of access. These issues can be resolved. British Columbia and Ontario have developed provincial capacity for planning, policy development and monitoring of children's mental health services – models are available. However, the pressure to make change does not appear to be present.

Nevertheless, it is heartening to note that the new hospital beds for youth mental health in Regina have been organized in partnership with the longstanding outpatient program of Regina Child and Youth Services. It is more usual in Canada to develop inpatient units for youth with a hospital focus separately from the outpatient programs resulting in unhealthy competition for resources and a distinct lack of cooperation at the clinical level. Without a common administration, it is very unlikely that the new inpatient unit would have been developed in partnership with the existing programs as has been done in Regina.

FUNDING MODELS

Throughout this document we have seen examples of program development or organization occurring to maximize the funding available. This is not a new phenomenon. To look back to the Saskatchewan history, during the 1960s when the Government of Canada indicated that psychiatric beds in general hospitals would be eligible for federal funding but such beds in mental hospitals would not be eligible, the Saskatchewan Plan for Mental Health with its regional mental hospitals soon metamorphosed into Saskatchewan Plan 2 – with psychiatric beds in general hospitals. When residential services for persons with a developmental disability became eligible for federal funding through Social Services departments in Saskatchewan a new agency, Core Services as part of the Ministry of Social Services, was created.

One hopes that the funding models are developed on the basis of good social policy for all and not solely with an eye to other objectives.

Health departments in Canadian provinces including Saskatchewan continue to favour fee for service physician payment rather than the development of a comprehensive and specialized interdisciplinary approach to the provision of services. This issue has been raised in various studies of health services – including in the Romanow Report which recommended a new approach to the delivery of primary health care. While there are hundreds of primary health care organizations in place across the country and numerous initiatives underway to create more, to quote Romanow

> "Unfortunately, for the most part, efforts made across Canada to implement primary health care have concentrated on isolated pilot projects with short-term funding".[164]

So the predominant model for physician funding remains as it has always been – fee for service.

Saskatchewan continues to provide increasing amounts of money to private practice physicians through the Medical Services Plan. The majority of these funds flow to physicians in general practice who have little specific training in mental health diagnoses and treatment. There is no incentive for private practice physicians to participate in program planning and they are rarely involved except at the level of provision of care.

For psychiatrists, the fee for service option encourages them to choose private practice rather than work in a children's mental health clinic. Psychiatrists are located almost always in the major cities resulting in poor access to Medical Services Plan funded specialized services in rural areas.

REASONS FOR OPTIMISM
INTERDEPARTMENTAL PLANNING

The principles that Russell and many others worked to introduce into service development can be seen in action within provinces and also at the national level. Various steps have been taken to respond to the need for comprehensive and multi-disciplinary services, an issue that has always bedevilled planners and providers of service. Interdepartmental planning has been one of the keys to improvement.

In the 1990s in all provinces, joint planning initiatives among the departments and agencies responsible for managing services to children and youth became fashionable. In June of 1993 an interdepartmental committee in Saskatchewan circulated a policy framework for improving the well-being of Saskatchewan's children titled *Children First*.[165] It was circulated to more than 1200 organizations and comments were requested. From this consultation they developed a children's agenda for the future – *Saskatchewan's Action Plan for Children – a Plan for Change*.[166]

The action plan has been operationalized and resulted in significant changes for the better. In 1994 an Office of the Children's Advocate associated with the Office of the Ombudsman was established and at the same time the Saskatchewan Council on Children was created as a forum for discussion and advice to government in all areas of community life as they impact upon young people. As well, over the next several years government funded a number of community initiatives focused on providing integrated services to youngsters and their families including integrated school-linked services, early intervention programs, the Family Law Division of the Court of Queen's Bench, and numerous Indian Child and Family Service agencies.

Saskatchewan's efforts on behalf of children were recognized by the Child Welfare League of Canada who conferred their award, Champions for Children, in 1996 on the province. The interdepartmental committee continues to provide leadership within government with the support of the Council. The concerns are wide-ranging and geared to strengthen families and communities to provide for children. An Early Childhood Development Strategy – Kids First, was an early success. The Role of Schools Review resulted in a new program thrust centred on the school as the hub for meeting the needs of youngsters. The Saskatchewan Council on Children has been renamed The Council on Children and Youth and will provide leadership in implementation of the SchoolPlus initiative.

The Interdepartmental Steering Committee responsible for Saskatchewan's Action Plan for Children has successfully kept the issues of children and youth on the agenda of government for a decade.

OFFICE OF THE OMBUDSMAN AND CHILDREN'S ADVOCATE

This document frequently bewails the lack of advocates for children and youth. There have traditionally been few avenues for children's voices to be heard and few people speaking on their behalf. In recent years the creation of Ombudsmen and Children's Advocates has helped to redress this situation.

During the last twenty-five years provinces have established Ombudsman Offices to act as an independent voice for citizens concerned with government services. Further, many provinces have established specialized organizations like the Saskatchewan Children's Advocate to act as a voice for children and promote their interests when there are concerns about government services. These offices investigate individual complaints and work with the complainant and the service provider to resolve the problem.

The Saskatchewan Children's Advocate Office authority is derived from the Ombudsman and Children's Advocate Act. As well as dealing with individual complaints the Children's Advocate has the authority to conduct systemic advocacy to promote and advocate for changes to government practice, policy or legislation respecting the interests and wellbeing of children. As well as advocating for change and public education the Children's Advocate may make formal recommendations to government departments and agencies.

The development of Ombudsman and Children's Advocate legislation at the provincial level has provided a formal way for citizens to express their concern about individual children or about the broader needs of a group or class of children. For the most part, children do not have the capacity to speak on their own behalf. This legislated form of public advocacy on behalf of children and youth provides a new voice on behalf of young people. Given that the Children's Advocate reports to the legislature, the voice of the advocate is heard by the politicians and as a consequence the likelihood of action for change is increased.

IT'S TIME FOR A PLAN FOR CHILDREN'S MENTAL HEALTH

Lack of planning and the consequence that children's mental health services 'just grew' has been an ongoing problem for many years. Now several provinces have comprehensive plans for children's mental health services.

In 2004 the Saskatchewan Children's Advocate produced *It's Time for a Plan for Children's Mental Health.*[167] The report summarized earlier recommendations made about mental health services and replies made by government officials. A vigorous case was made to change the system of services to create a new service delivery capacity that employs state of the art, evidence-based practices and accountability for outcomes.

The report was "intended to provide a catalyst for action to create a comprehensive plan to ensure adequate and appropriate children's mental health services throughout the province". The lack of a clear direction and plan for service provision and development was described as a major barrier to adequate mental health services. The recommendation generated by the report is clear:

> "That Saskatchewan Health, in consultation with stakeholders, develop and implement a comprehensive plan to ensure that mental health services are provided to Saskatchewan children, youth and families in a manner that is consistent with what is known about best practices."

The government through Saskatchewan Health did act on the recommendation of the Children's Advocate and a Plan for Child and Youth Mental Health Services[168] was released in 2007.

British Columbia had been the first province to develop a plan with their February 2003 *BC Child and Youth Metal Health Plan*[169]. It was a five-year plan and provided leadership within the province. During the term of the plan significant budget, program and staff enhancements have been made. At the conclusion of the five years a review was commissioned which reported that while there were a number of successes, that much work remained to be done.[170] Alberta has more recently announced a ten-year report and framework for child and youth mental health 2006-2016.[171]

In 2007, The Canadian Paediatric Society called upon the federal government to develop a national and coordinated strategy for mental illness and mental health that includes a specific focus on children and youth. They also urged each provincial and territorial government to develop and implement a mental health care plan for children and youth. They rated each province and territory on their current plans. At the time of writing, only four provinces had a current plan specific to child and youth mental health although other jurisdictions included children in their mental health plan or in their child health plan.[172]

In August 2007 Prime Minister Harper announced the

membership of a national Mental Health Commission. One of its advisory committees will be a children's and youth advisory committee and one of its key initiatives has been identified as the promotion of the development of a national strategy. This will be watched with great interest.

THE RECENT HISTORY OF GOVERNMENT INTERVENTIONISM

The creation of responsibility centres within provincial governments has helped to improve interdepartmental planning and public advocacy.

The International Year of the Child 1979 marked the beginning of many important changes in Canadian society on behalf of children and youth. The most tangible legacy has been the establishment within governments of responsibility centres for children and youth. This has been the result of the efforts of public advocacy movements to keep children on the political agenda. The establishment of these responsibility centres within provincial governments has improved coordination and provided a higher profile for children's services. The traditions in Canada of social advocacy movements and strong public service planning have been reinforced by these moves. These responsibility centres have taken various forms in different jurisdictions. However, it is clear to all governments in Canada that the needs of children, youth and families must be addressed. Children and youth are on the political agenda and have been addressed in a variety of ways by provincial governments:

- By consolidating all services for the young in a single government department that is responsible for planning, funding and service delivery;

- By establishing government secretariats that are coalitions of departments or ministries charged with the responsibility of coordinating service planning, funding and delivery;

- By formalizing action plans that focus on government priorities and funding to ensure that children receive a fair share of policy attention and resources;

- By creating offices of ombudsman for children, child advocates or other independent offices to investigate and advocate on behalf of the needs of youngsters;

- By establishing royal commissions or independent mechanisms to investigate the needs of children and youth and make recommendations for change; and

- By funding national and provincial strategies to address major problems such as alcohol and drug abuse, family violence, child sexual abuse, school dropouts, youth unemployment, environmental protection and youth involvement, childcare, and poverty.

Canadians expect their governments and politicians to be responsive. Advocacy on behalf of the young at the personal, community and government levels continues to be needed as it is a powerful influence on decision-makers.

The governance and delivery of services for children and youth is primarily the responsibility of the provinces with the federal role limited for the most part to the collection of taxes and agreements for the transfer of funds to the provinces. The needs of the young have been studied and debated nationally, provincially and locally by government and citizen advocacy groups over the years. Service delivery systems are constantly evolving to better meet the needs of the vulnerable young and their families. Recent directions to improve services to children and youth have included:

- movement towards coordinated planning structures in government,

- integrating various services into common management structures,

- increased local or regional autonomy to deliver services, and creation of specialized watchdog functions such as children's ombudsman, children's advocate or commissioners.

CONCLUSION

There have been significant improvements in the system of services for children and youth over the last forty years. The resource base has been considerably enhanced. Integration of children with special needs into mainstream programs has been and continues to be a priority. Program and professional specialization has increased and serves to meet the needs of the majority of youngsters. The recognition of the importance of the wider problems of social and economic disparity are being addressed, especially through early childhood development programs at the community level, many of which are focused on the needs of youngsters in Aboriginal communities. While children still do not have a voice in debates on social policy, the interests and needs of children are increasingly recognized in decisions made on their behalf.

While Chapter 1 began with a quotation from a 2006 Senate report that characterized children's mental health services as 'the orphan's orphan' within the health care system, there have been many improvements in the past 40 years.

As well as the initiatives identified above there have been major funding increases for children's mental health services in several provinces. The development of outcome measures is moving ahead in some areas, British Columbia for one, and program evaluation is a term being heard more often. We are still a long way from a situation where every child has access to the mental health services the child may need and there will no doubt be many more growing pains as services develop and expand. We owe it to our children to continue the development of mental health services for children and youth to meet their needs in the twenty-first century.

Afterword

By 2004 Child and Youth Services had once again outgrown its space and moved to expanded quarters at Albert St and 10th Avenue in downtown Regina. For the first time in its history the program had purpose-designed space and sufficient offices and amenities for its growing clientele and staff.

In 2011 Regina Child and Youth Services had 73 positions including psychologists, social workers, psychiatric and registered nurses, occupational therapists, speech-language pathologists, child psychiatrists, a developmental paediatrician and administrative staff. It had an annual budget of over $9 million and had an average active caseload of over 2200 cases.

As it has from its beginning, the same principles underlie the programs. Regina Child and Youth Services is part of a comprehensive program that includes services ranging from health promotion to residential care. It offers a multi-disciplinary clinical approach where professionals from many disciplines bring their particular skills to assessment and treatment.

It is a regional program with services delivered close to the person's home and family. And it uses a community building approach, working together on behalf of other systems, providing consultation and assisting them to address problems. Services are family centred – reflecting the conviction that support to the family is a primary means of assisting their child. And early intervention is always a priority.

MILESTONES

ADOLESCENT SEXUAL OFFENDERS PROGRAM

In 1989 through a province-wide Cabinet initiative two staff were designated to develop a new Adolescent Sexual Offenders Program at RCYS. Building on the cooperative relationship already established with the Regina Young Offender Program they developed an assessment process and a new case management approach. Early experimentation with separate psycho-educational classes for parents and youth proved successful and is used along with group and individual therapy. This specialized program accepts many referrals from outside the Regina region and program staff provides training and consultation to workers in other systems and other regions.

THE ALLIANCE FOR SUICIDE AWARENESS AND PREVENTION (ASAP)

In 1991, following a high-profile youth suicide in Regina, Child and Youth Services initiated a series of community stakeholder meetings to discuss options to address the problem of youth suicide. The Adolescent Suicide Awareness and Prevention Program (ASAP) was established as an advisory council to support community partnerships, to train front line workers in suicide prevention, to provide consultation to enhance and support needed by persons at risk, to raise community awareness, and to develop protocols to provide appropriate service after an event. By 1999 ASAP had trained over 800 professionals and other caregivers through a certified Suicide Intervention Workshop. Saskatchewan Health funded new suicide prevention positions for each mental health region in 1996 and the Regina program has since expanded its mandate to include broad prevention programming for the entire region.

THE RANDALL KINSHIP CENTRE

The Kinship Centre opened in 2002 as a satellite location of RCYS. It was named after David Randall, the RCYS director at the time. The program was developed to meet the needs of families with children and youth who have very disruptive behavioural problems. Many of the young people are aboriginal and half of the staff are First Nations or Métis social workers. The whole family is the focus of treatment and support. Services are staffed and provided in a way that honours First Nations and Métis cultures, values and beliefs. The team has provided leadership in developing a culturally affirming workplace. A group of staff comprise the Cultural Brokers who organize training, feasts, celebrations for National Aboriginal Day and other occasions. First Nations Elders provide advice to clinicians, work directly with families and provide training on First Nations teachings. The Kinship Centre also is responsible to provide Community Parent Education, an evidence based parenting program for children with disruptive behavior. This is offered in partnership with the two Regina school boards. A wide range of programs are provided; parenting education, crisis services and care delivered in the home and neighbourhood. Special programs are available for Aboriginal Problem Gambling and Addiction Problems of Young Offenders. Group services are offered to youth through Double Trouble -- an eight-week program for youth who harmfully use substances and may have a concurrent mental health diagnosis. These young people are either at risk of becoming involved or are currently involved in the youth criminal justice system.

TOUCHSTONE PROGRAM

The federal government funds a treatment program for high risk violent offenders who are usually incarcerated at a young offender's facility.

ADOLESCENT PSYCHIATRY UNIT

In 2004 the management of the Regina General Hospital's Medical Adolescent Unit was assumed by the Mental Health and Addictions Branch of the health region. This is a 10 bed unit for youth age 11 to 18 and is managed by a senior psychologist at RCYS. The child psychiatrists employed by RCYS admit and treat short term acutely ill young people. The planning for the unit also includes a community outreach component that will link a number of existing community-based youth services and build supports to keep youth in the community while receiving mental health care.

KIDS FIRST MENTAL HEALTH/ADDICTIONS TEAM

This is a community-based program directed by a community board and provides early intervention to vulnerable expectant and new mothers and their children to age 5. The families are identified in hospital and the program is a home visiting early intervention model. The Kids First Mental Health team consults to the home visitors who are paraprofessional, provide training to them and assess children who require additional services.

COGNITIVE DISABILITIES ASSESSMENT PROGRAM

This program provides assessment and diagnosis to children and young adults age 6 to 24, primarily those with fetal alcohol syndrome disorder. Consultation, training and direct services are provided to three other southern health regions.

AUTISM SERVICES

Following a 2007 external review Regina Child and Youth Services developed a three-year project to improve autism services. In 2010 the provincial government announced $2.5 million for enhanced services with $1.1 million targeted for Regina and surrounding areas. Now all diagnosis and services to children are the responsibility of Child and Youth Services while the Autism Resource Centre provides care to adults with autism. Services provided by Child and Youth Services include case management, service providers for some clients including all preschoolers, skill development groups, parent training groups and respite.

EARLY PSYCHOSIS

In 2007 Saskatchewan unveiled a Mental Health Plan for Children and Youth. It included funding for three positions to Regina Child and Youth Services to provide differential diagnosis and assertive case management to youth and young adults, age 14 to 30 who are psychotic. This is an assertive outreach program which also provides distance consultation. Much of the distance consultation is done through telehealth.

INTERNSHIPS AND PRACTICA

Expanding upon a practice begun many years ago, students from a variety of disciplines regularly gain work experience at CYS as part of their training. As well, Child and Youth Services is now an accredited site for PhD Psychology internships.

CONSULTATIONS AND PARTNERSHIPS

Along with formal consulting arrangements with twenty community child serving programs, CYS has partnerships with both Regina School Boards and with Ehrlo Community Services. This latter partnership enables CYS to provide a range of group activities – sports and arts/crafts -- to focus on social skills development and provide respite to parents. Child and Youth Services also participates on many inter-sectoral committees.

There are evening hours two evenings a week and programs on both Saturdays and Sundays. RCYS offered 38 different therapy groups in 2011.

Notes

1   Understanding Mental Health and Mental Health Services

1   Government of Canada Standing Senate Committee on Social Affairs, Science and Technology Out of the Shadows at Last. Kirby 2006.

2   Federal/Provincial/Territorial Advisory Committee on the Mental Health of Children and Youth. 1990. Foundations for the Future, Health Canada, Ottawa.

3   Ibid.

4   Government of Canada. 1964. Mental Health for Canadians: Striking a Balance, Department of National Health and Welfare, Ottawa.

5   Waddell C., Offord DR, Shepherd CA, Hua JM and McEwan K. 2002, Child Psychiatric Epidemiology and Canadian Public Policy-Making: The State of Science and the Art of the Possible. Canadian Journal of Psychiatry. 2002.47(9): 825-832.

6   Sun Life Financial Chair on Adolescent Mental Health Backgrounder October 2006.

7   Government of British Columbia 2003 BC Child and Youth Mental Health Plan. Victoria.

8   Sun Life Financial Chair on Adolescent Mental Health Backgrounder October 2006.

9   Foundations for the Future, 1990.

10   Jones, K. 1999. Taming the Troublesome Child: American Families, Child Guidance, and the Limits of Psychiatric Authority. Harvard University Press, Cambridge, Ma.

11   Lourie, Ira S. 2003. A History of Community Child Mental Health. In A.J. Pumariega and N.C. Winters (Eds.). The Handbook of Child and Adolescent Systems of Care. John Wiley & Sons, San Francisco.

12   Pumariega, AJ & Winters, NC. 2003. The Handbook of Child and Adolescent Systems of Care, Jossey-Bass, A Wiley Imprint, San Francisco.

13   Government of Ontario, 1968-69. Children's Mental Health Centres Act. Revised 1976. Toronto.

14   Government of Alberta. 1985. The Child and Family Services Act. Edmonton.

15   Uniform Law Conference. 1987. Uniform Mental Health Act, Government of Canada, Ottawa.

16   Government of Canada. 1984. Young Offender's Act. Ottawa

17   Canadian Council on Children and Youth. 1978. Admittance Restricted: The Child as Citizen in Canada, M.O.M. Printing, Ottawa.

18   Russell, T. 1996. Guiding Principles for Mental Health Services for Children and Youth, Canada's Children, Journal of the Child Welfare League of Canada, Vol 3.

19   Government of Great Britain. 1867. British North America Act. London.

20   Government of Canada. 1982. Canadian Constitution, Ottawa.

21   Russel, T. and Pearson, L. 1983. Voluntary Organizations and Child Welfare Policy, in Social Work Papers, Volume 17.

22   Zachik, A, Heffron, W, Junek, W and Russell, T. 2003 Relationships Between Systems of Care and Federal, State and Local Governments. In Pumariega, A and Winters, N. Eds. The Handbook of Child and Adolescent Systems of Care, John Wiley & Sons, San Francisco.

23   Government of Canada. 1984. Canada Health Act, Ottawa.

24   Government of Canada. 1966 Canada Assistance Plan, Ottawa.

25   Government of Canada. 1996 Canada Health and Social Transfer Program. Ottawa.

26   Children's Mental Health Centres Act. Revised 1976.

27   The Child and Family Services Act. Edmonton. 1985.

2   The Context – the National Scene to 1985

28   Law Reform Commission on Children's and Family Law, Victoria.

29   Saskatchewan Law Reform Commission. 1976. Children's Maintenance. Government of Saskatchewan, Regina.

30   Canadian Council on Children and Youth. 1984. Synopsis of Recommendations Drawn from the Report of the Committee on Sexual Offences Against Children. Ottawa.

31   United Nation Declaration on the Rights of the Child. 1989 PD-UN.

32   Children's Maintenance. 1976.

33   Admittance Restricted: The Child as Citizen in Canada Canadian Council on Children and Youth. 1981.

34   Children and Culture in Canada. Research paper submitted to the Federal Cultural Policy Review Committee. Ottawa.

35   Canadian Council on Children and Youth. 1984. Media Kit on the Committee on Sexual Offences Against Children. Ottawa.

36   Admittance Restricted: The Child as Citizen in Canada

37   Ibid.

38   Haines, E.H. 1976-77. The use of expert assistance in disputed custody cases. Family Law Practice Notes, Ontario Bar Commission. Toronto.

39   Commission on Emotional and Learning Disorders in Children, One Million Children – the CELDIC Report, Toronto, 1970.

40   Interdepartmental Coordinating Committee on Rehabilitation. 1964. Services to Emotionally Disturbed Children in Saskatchewan: Committee Report and Recommendations. Government of Saskatchewan. Regina.

41   Kempe, C., Silverman, F., Steele, B., Droegmueller, W. & Silver, H. 1962. The Battered Child Syndrome. Journal of the American Medical Association, 181, 17-24.

42   Van Stolk, M., 1972. The Battered Child in Canada, Toronto: McClelland and Stewart Ltd.

43   Government of Canada, House of Commons Standing Committee on Health, Welfare and Social Affairs. 1976. Proceedings Ottawa.

44   Committee on Sexual Offences Against Children. Sexual Offences Against Children, Volumes 1 and 2. Supply and Services Canada, Ottawa, 1984.

45   Rogers, Rix. 1990. Reaching for Solutions, Health Canada, Ottawa.

46   For Canada's Children: National Agenda for Action.

47   Pearson, Landon. 1980. Introduction to For Canada's Children: National Agenda for Action. Canadian Commission on the International Year of the Child, Ottawa.

48   For Canada's Children: National Agenda for Action.

49   Cruickshank, D. et al. 1980. Minutes and Proceedings, Joint Committee of the Senate and House of Commons on the Constitution of Canada. Ottawa.

50   Government of Canada. 1908. The Juvenile Delinquent's Act. Ottawa.

51   Lane, K. 1995. The Philosophy of the Young Offenders Act and Its Impact on the Formal Legal Education and Practice Advocates for Youth, LLM Thesis, University of Alberta, Edmonton.

52   Government of Canada. 1995. Young Offenders Act. Ottawa.

53   Government of Canada. 2002. Youth Criminal Justice Act. Ottawa.

54   Anand, S. Quoted in Green R. & Hurley, K. Tough on Kids, p. 48. Purich Publishing Limited, Saskatoon, 2003.

3   The Mental Hospital Years

55   Johnson, AW. Dream No Little Dreams, A Biography of the Douglas Government of Saskatchewan, 1944-1961:University of Toronto Press,2004.

56   Statutes of Canada, Chapter 51, Sections 10-13. 1885 Ottawa.

57   Government of Saskatchewan. 1906. The Insanity Act. Regina.

58   Government of Saskatchewan. Department of Public Works, Memo Re: Asylum, 1906.

59   The Insanity Act. 1906.

60   Low, D. 1907. Commissioner's Report to the Province of Saskatchewan. Government of Saskatchewan, Regina.

61   Government of Saskatchewan, 1906, 1916, 1917, 1933, 1923, 1924. Department of Public Works Annual Reports. Regina.

62   Government of Saskatchewan. 1914. Act to Appoint an Administrator of Lunatics' Estates. Regina.

63   Government of Saskatchewan, 1906, 1916, 1917, 1933, 1923, 1924. Department of Public Works Annual Reports. Regina.

64   Ibid.

65   Government of Saskatchewan. 1917. Inspector's Report by Gerhard Enns, MLA for Rosthern. Regina.

66   Government of Saskatchewan, 1906, 1916, 1917, 1933, 1923, 1924. Department of Public Works Annual Reports. Regina.

67   Ibid.

68   Ibid.

69   Government of Saskatchewan, 1906, 1916, 1917, 1922, 1933, 1923, 1924. Department of Public Works Annual Reports.

70   Ibid.

71   Saskatchewan Health. 1980. Saskatchewan Health for Children and Youth. Regina.

72   Saskatchewan Health for Children and Youth.

73   Government of Saskatchewan. 1925. Annual Report of the Deputy Minister of Public Health, Regina.

74   Hincks, C. 1930. Provincial Mental Hospitals and Mental Hygiene Conditions in the Province of Saskatchewan. Government of Saskatchewan. Regina.

75   Hincks, C. 1937. Facts and Observations Pertaining to the Mental Hygiene Situation in Saskatchewan. Government of Saskatchewan, Regina.

76   Johnson, A.W. Dream No Little Dreams, A Biography of the Douglas Government of Saskatchewan, 1944-1961: University of Toronto Press, 2004.

77   Lipset, S. 1968. Agrarian Socialism: The Cooperative Commonwealth Federation in Saskatchewan. Anchor Books,

78   Liberty Magazine. 1947. Canada's Shame: Our Mental Hospitals, February 8.

79   Hincks, C. 1945. Mental Hygiene Survey of Saskatchewan. Government of Saskatchewan, Regina.

80   Dickinson, Harley D. 1989. The Two Psychiatries: The Transformation of Psychiatric Work in Saskatchewan, Canadian Plains Research Centre, University of Regina, 1989.

81   Mills, John. "Lessons from the periphery: psychiatry in Saskatchewan, Canada, 1944-68" in History of Psychiatry 18(2): 179-201.

82   The Two Psychiatries: The Transformation of Psychiatric Work in Saskatchewan.

83   "Lessons from the periphery: psychiatry in Saskatchewan, Canada, 1944-68".

84   Ibid., 1944-68.

85   Ibid., 1944-68.

86   Smith, C., 'Crisis and Aftermath', Canadian Psychiatric Association Journal, February 1971.

4   Setting the Stage

87   Government of Saskatchewan. 1953. Department of Public Health Annual Report. Regina.

88   The Two Psychiatries: The Transformation of Psychiatric Work in Saskatchewan.

89   Laycock, SR. 1930. Commissioner's Report on Mental Hygiene Conditions, Government of Saskatchewan.

90   Treherne, D. 1984. Educational Psychology in Saskatchewan: A Review of its History and Current Directions, Saskatchewan Psychologist, Vol 84/Number 2/May 1984.

91   Griffin, J.D.M., Laycock, S.R. & Line, W. 1940. Manual for Teachers: Mental Hygiene, University of Toronto.

92   Interdepartmental Coordinating Committee on Rehabilitation. Committee Report and Recommendations: Services to Emotionally Disturbed Children in Saskatchewan. 1964.

93   Pawson, G. & Russell, T. 1985. The Practice of Community Work in Child Welfare. In Theory and Practice of Community Social Work. S. Taylor & R. Roberts, Eds, Columbia University Press, New York.

94   Smith, C. 1973. A Decade of Psychiatry in Saskatchewan. Regina, Unpublished.

95   Bell, G. & Lafave, H. 1978. Children and Parents: Changing Services in a Changing World. Paper presented at the International Association of Child Psychiatry and Allied Professions, 9th International Congress, Melbourne.

96   Frazier, S.H. & Pokorny, A.D. 1968. Report of a Consultation to the Minister of Public Health on Psychiatric Services in Saskatchewan. Department of Public Health, Regina.

97   The Two Psychiatries: The Transformation of Psychiatric Work in Saskatchewan.

98   Report of a Consultation to the Minister of Public Health on Psychiatric Services in Saskatchewan.

99   Gauthier, Y. 1969. Child and Family Mental Health Services: Future Policy Issues, Canada's Mental Health, 26, 1, p2.

100   The Two Psychiatries: The Transformation of Psychiatric Work in Saskatchewan.

101   Russell, T. 1976. Responsibility for the Handicapped Child. The School Trustee, V. XXIX, No. 1.

102   Government of Saskatchewan. 1971. The School Act. Regina.

103   The Practice of Community Work in Child Welfare.

5   The Beginnings of a New Program

104   Russell, T. 1970. The Role of the Psychiatric Services Branch in Services to Children and Youth: With Special Reference to the Needs in Regina, Unpublished.

105   Asselstine, J. 1971. Three Year Development Plan for Services to Children and Adolescents, Report commissioned by Department of Public Health, Psychiatric Services Branch, Regina.

106   The Two Psychiatries: The Transformation of Psychiatric Work in Saskatchewan.

107   Psychiatric Services Branch. 1972. Ad Hoc Committee on Psychiatric Team Structure. Saskatchewan Health, Regina.

108   Smith, C. 1974. Memo to all Staff from Director of Psychiatric Services Branch Re: Role of Paramedical Professions, Psychiatric Services Branch, Regina.

109   Smith, C., Memo to W. Shmishek, Minister of Health re: Psychiatric Referrals. Psychiatric Services Branch, Regina, 1972.

110   Russell, T. 1974. The Development of Consultative Mental Health Services to Children and Families. Psychiatric Services Branch, Regina.

111   Treherne, D., Russell, T. & Kelly, D. 1974. Problems with the Provision of Services to Children and Adolescents in Saskatchewan, Report to the Thrust Committee of the Department of Public Health.

112   The Development of Consultative Mental Health Services to Children and Families.

113   One Million Children – the CELDIC Report.

114   Committee Report and Recommendations: Services to Emotionally Disturbed Children in Saskatchewan.

115   Three Year Development Plan for Services to Children and Adolescents.

116   The Two Psychiatries: The Transformation of Psychiatric Work in Saskatchewan.

117   The Development of Consultative Mental Health Services to Children and Families.

118   Russell, T. & Bell, G. 1975. The Provision of Mental Health Services to Children and Families, Western Canadian Study Session on Human Services to Rural Communities, Banff.

119   The Provision of Mental Health Services to Children and Families 1975.

120   Bell, G. & Russell, T. 1975. Organizational Models of Health Service Delivery. Paper presented at the Western Canadian Study Session on Human Services to Rural Communities, Banff.

121   Bell, G. 1978. Interim Report of the Child and Youth Services Advisory Committee, Psychiatric Services Branch, Saskatchewan Health, Regina.

122   Saskatchewan Health. 1980. Current Health Resources, Organization and Utilization. Regina.

6   Regina Child and Youth Services 1968-88

123   Hogan, E. 1968. Memo re: Munroe Wing – Children's Clinic, to Dr. J.A. Chapman, Director, Munroe Wing and Clinic. Regina.

124   The Two Psychiatries: The Transformation of Psychiatric Work in Saskatchewan.

125   Russell, T. 1972. Children from Rural Areas Registered at Harding House. Memo to Joe Dvernichuk, Associate Director, Psychiatric Services Branch.

126   Elias, J. 1974. Program Analysis of Harding House, PASS Analysis, Department of Public Health.

127   The Development of Consultative Mental Health Services to Children and Families.

128   Smith, C. 1974. Memo to all Staff from Director of Psychiatric Services Branch Re: Role of Paramedical Professions, Psychiatric Services Branch, Regina.

129   The Two Psychiatries: The Transformation of Psychiatric Work in Saskatchewan.

130   Children and Parents: Changing Services in a Changing World.

131   Ibid.

132   Beck, Marion. Ed. 1977. 1977. Proceedings of the First National Conference: Autism the Whole Spectrum. Canadian Society for Autistic Children. Regina.

7   International Year of the Child and International Year of Youth

133   Saskatchewan Health. 1980. Current Health Resources, Organization and Utilization. Regina.

134   Saskatchewan Health. 1980. Youth, Health and Lifestyles Regina.

135   Saskatchewan Health. 1984. Learning Through Living Health. Regina.

136   Saskatchewan Health for Children and Youth. Regina.

137   Saskatchewan Health. 1980. Minister's Speaking Notes on the Release of the Review of Child Health Services. Regina.

138   Saskatchewan Health, 1981, January 9. Memorandum from Ken Fyke, Deputy Minister, Re: Joint Task Force on Services to Children and Youth. Regina.

139   Saskatchewan Health. 1981. Child Health Joint Task Force Report. Regina.

140   Child Health Joint Task Force Report.

141   Kent, E. 1981. Memo Re: Child Health. Department of Health. Regina.

156 Junek, RW. & Thompson, AH. 1996. Self-regulating Service Delivery Systems: A model for Children and Youth at Risk. Journal of Behavioural Health Services and Research, 26, 64-79.

157 Doherty, G. 1985. Provision of Services to Children with Behavioural or Emotional Problems, Alberta Social Services and Community Health, 1985.

158 Campbell, P. and Thompson, A. 1988. Provision of Services to Children with Behavioural or Emotional Problems: An update of Provincial Services. Report commissioned by the Federal/Provincial/Territorial Committee on Mental Health Services for Children and Youth.

159 Russell,T. 2000. Inventory of Mental Health and Related Services in Canada. Childhood and Youth Division, Population Health Branch, Health Canada, Ottawa.

160 Provision of Services to Children with Behavioural or Emotional Problems.

161 Inventory of Mental Health and Related Services in Canada.

162 Ibid.

10   Moving Ahead

163 Carment, L. 1987. The Effects of Budget Restrictions. Report prepared for a meeting with the Deputy Minister of Health. Russell Papers.

164 Commission on the Future of Health Care in Canada, Building on Values: The Future of Health Care in Canada – Final Report. National Library of Canada 2002.

165 Government of Saskatchewan. 1993. Children First: An Invitation to Work Together – Creating Saskatchewan's Action Plan for Children. Regina.

166 Government of Saskatchewan. 1997. Our Children, Our Future: Saskatchewan's Action Plan for Children – Four Years Later. Regina.

167 Saskatchewan Children's Advocate. 2004. It's Time for a Plan for Children's Mental Health. Government of Saskatchewan. Regina.

168 Saskatchewan Health. A Better Future for Youth; Saskatchewan's Plan for Child & Youth Mental Health Services. Regina. 2005-6.

169 Government of British Columbia. The B.C. Child and Youth Mental Health Plan 2003. Ministry of Children and Family Development and Ministry of Health Services Joint Working Group. Victoria.

170 Berland, A. 2008. A Review of Child and Youth Mental Health Services in BC following implementation of the 2003 Child and Youth Mental Health Plan. Prepared for the Ministry of Children and Family Development. Victoria.

171 Government of Alberta. 2006. The Policy Framework: Mental Health for Alberta's Children and Youth.

172 Canadian Paediatric Society. Are We Doing Enough? A status report on Canadian public policy and child and youth health. Ottawa Ont.

Index

www.ingramcontent.com/pod-product-compliance
Lightning Source LLC
Chambersburg PA
CBHW070910270326
41927CB00011B/2515